Sex

AN EROTIC JOURNAL FOR SEXUAL INSPIRATION AND EXPLORATION

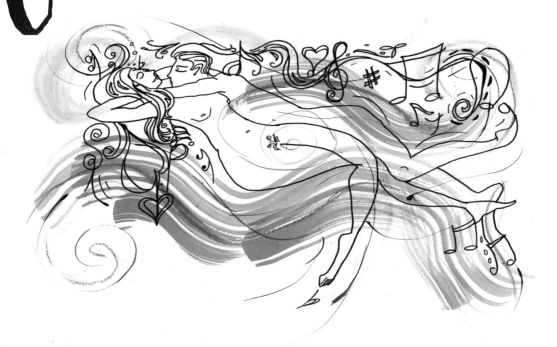

Illustrations by Margaret Hurst
with Jordan LaRousse

Kissing

What makes a good kisser? The cliché phrase "It takes two to tango" really applies here because a good kiss literally depends on the chemistry between two people. In fact when a woman kisses a man, part of the reason that she becomes aroused is because she is absorbing his testosterone through her mucus membranes. The more testosterone your man has to share, the hornier you'll feel!

DESCRIBE IN DETAIL your most memorable kiss. What made it so special? Who was the kisser? Do you recall the shape of his or her lips? Did he have stubble or a beard? Or was she smooth and soft? Where were you, and how old were you? Record as many sensations, scents, feelings, or emotions around this kiss as you can remember.

_____

_____

_____

_____

_____

_____

_____

_____

_____

_____

_____

"You should be kissed and often, and by someone who knows how."
—MARGARET MITCHELL, *GONE WITH THE WIND*

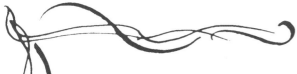

IN THE SPIRIT of Andy Warhol, create a sequence of kiss imprints in a pop-art style. (Think Warhol's famous *Marilyn* or *Campbell's Soup Cans*). Don a variety of lipstick colors, and kiss a piece of paper between each color change. Or get really creative: Using origami or wrapping paper, make a series of lips cut out of different paper colors and paste them to a poster board. If you want to go authentic Warhol style, use acrylic paint to reproduce your lips! Send your lips to your special someone, or make a series inspired by your lover's (or lovers') lips to keep for yourself!

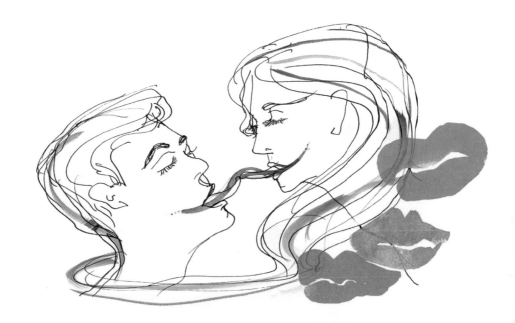

What Foreplay Means to Me

Foreplay can incorporate so many different things, from a sexy night out on the town to exchanging erotic emails while at work. Use these pages to explore what amazing foreplay means to you.

FIRST, WRITE DOWN what typical foreplay is like for you. For example, "Usually, we start caressing each other under the bed covers, we get naked, my partner goes down on me, I go down on him, and then sex begins." Now, shatter this notion of boring same ol' same ol' foreplay and write down a sexy scenario that would *really* get you hot and bothered. For example, "While we're both still at work, my partner starts by texting me naughty ideas he's been having about tying me up and spanking me." Try to think of several elements to your new foreplay script that go against your normal routine, and that would truly turn you on.

_____

_____

_____

_____

_____

_____

_____

_____

_____

_____

_____

_____

_____

"I'm a foreplay junkie." — RICHARD DREYFUSS, AMERICAN ACTOR

PUT THE *play* **INTO FOREPLAY**. It's time to design a little foreplay game of your own. What you'll need: a stack of twenty medium-size notecards (blank with no lines), a three-minute timer (you can use the one on your phone), and a partner. On each of the twenty note cards, draw an image and a short written cue of what you'd like for your partner to do to you or what you'd like to do to them—make sure the activities are foreplay and don't involve penetration. Ideas include kissing, foot massage, head massage, touching specific areas of the body, and sex talk. Shuffle the cards and put them facedown in a stack. One by one, draw the cards and act out the image or directions on the card with your partner. Set the timer and engage in the foreplay act until the time runs out before choosing a new card. See how turned on you feel by the time you've gotten through the deck.

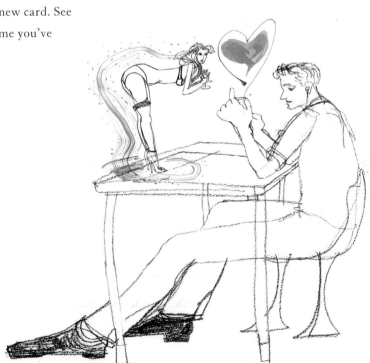

How Many Minutes Does It Take To . . . ?

Ladies, set your timers
and get to know your
pleasure cycle. By
learning how long it
takes for your body to
respond to sexual
stimuli, you'll know
more about yourself.

"Sex: the thing that takes up the least amount of time and causes the most amount of trouble." —JOHN BARRYMORE, EARLY TWENTIETH-CENTURY AMERICAN ACTOR

Speaking of time, there's a fun product on the market called Little Rooster. It's a vibrating alarm clock that you wear on your pubic region while you sleep. At the preset time, it sends gentle vibrations to your clitoris so that you wake up in response to feelings of pleasure, rather than the blaring of a traditional alarm clock. Now that's a great wake-up call! Check it out at littleroosterstore.com.

1. TIME YOURSELF MASTURBATING. Use just your hands at first. Write down how long it takes for you (in minutes) to achieve orgasm from start to finish. Rate the quality of your orgasm from 0 to 10: 0 meaning you didn't have one and 10 meaning it was the best orgasm of your life.

_____

_____

_____

2. NOW TIME YOURSELF masturbating using your favorite sex aid and record the results as described above.

_____

_____

_____

3. IF YOU HAVE A WILLING PARTNER, set a timer to your next sexy play session. Press start from the moment of first penetration (with tongue, finger, penis, or toy). Record the results as described above, but this time also describe how excited your partner makes you and the scenario you were in. For example, was it a typical bedroom encounter? Or, were you on an exciting weekend getaway?

_____

_____

_____

_____

_____

Amazing Massage

A sexy massage does wonders to create a sensual mood. It is relaxing, can help alleviate stress, and stimulate your biggest organ . . . your skin. Use these pages to explore your experience being the recipient of a lover's massaging touch.

The most amazing massages take place outdoors: There is something very titillating about being nude, oiled, and rubbed while in the embrace of the sun's warm rays and surrounded by the sounds of birds, a river, or ocean waves. Make a sacred massage space somewhere outdoors where you can enjoy the beauty of a sensual massage. Set up a soft beach towel or blanket in a private location; this could be in your own backyard, on a porch, at a beach, or outside a forest cabin.

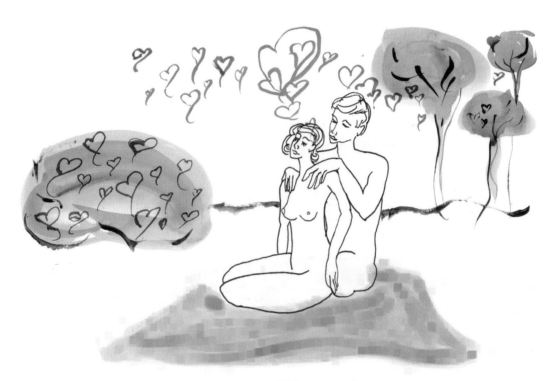

"I love a good massage, and they gotta go deep."
—ZOE LISTER-JONES, AMERICAN ACTRESS

BEFORE YOU RECEIVE a sexy massage, mentally scan your body from top to bottom and inside and out. Write down at least ten ways you feel. Think about how you feel both physically and emotionally (e.g., "Right shoulder is achy," "feeling tired"). After doing your scan, ask for a massage from your lover. Make sure he or she gives you his or her full attention and leaves no inch of your skin untouched. After the massage experience, again scan your body and write down ten to fifteen ways you feel physically and emotionally (e.g., "horny," "relaxed," "gooey," "The pain in my right shoulder is gone!"). Has your overall state of well-being improved? Describe the differences in the way you feel before and after the massage.

_____

_____

_____

_____

_____

_____

_____

_____

_____

_____

_____

_____

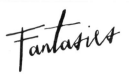

Fantasies

Our brains are our most powerful sexual organs. So it's not surprising that engaging in sexual fantasies is a powerful form of foreplay. Use these pages to explore your hidden desires.

WRITE A DESCRIPTION of a sexual fantasy that you have kept a secret from your partner or yourself. Spare no details. Use the opposite page to sketch your fantasy.

Having trouble uncovering your sexual fantasy? Try this game to get you started. Write down the following:

~

Your top three (or more!) sexy fantasy partners. They can be anyone in the world: a coworker, a movie star, or even your husband.

~

Now choose a partner from the above list (or all three?) and answer this: Who's in charge?

~

Select a fantasy location for you and your partner(s) to play. Are you in a mountain cabin? On a beach? Outside in the rain? In a movie theater?

~

Are there toys, lingerie, or props involved? Be specific.

~

Now play out the fantasy from beginning to end. How do you and your partner(s) encounter each other? What are you wearing, and what is he wearing? How does the fantasy scenario progress from encounter to sex? Have fun! This is your fantasy. There are no right or wrong answers.

"In my sex fantasy, nobody ever loves me for my mind."
—NORA EPHRON, AMERICAN JOURNALIST

My Ideal Lover

You've probably thought about your ideal lover before. Maybe it's a man who looks like Channing Tatum, or maybe it's a gorgeous woman who isn't afraid to call the shots in bed. Maybe you're lucky enough to be married to your ideal lover, or maybe your ideal is having a man in every port. You can learn a lot about yourself by investigating your personal concept of a perfect lover, whatever that may be.

WRITE DOWN the traits of your ideal lover. Use these prompts to get you started:

"My ideal lover isn't afraid to . . ."

_____

_____

_____

"My ideal lover looks like . . ."

_____

_____

_____

"My ideal lover works as a . . ."

_____

_____

_____

"My ideal lover gives me . . ."

_____

_____

_____

"My ideal lover makes me feel like . . ."

_____

_____

_____

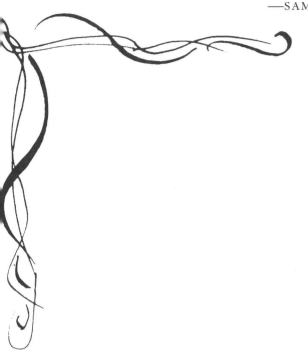

*"We come to love not by finding a perfect person,
but by learning to see an imperfect person perfectly."*
—SAM KEEN, FROM *TO LOVE AND BE LOVED*

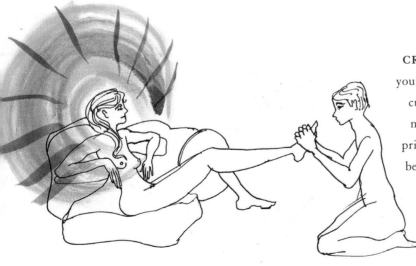

CREATE A COLLAGE of
your ideal lover's attributes by
cutting out photos from a
magazine or from online
printouts. Don't be afraid to
be as precise or as poetic as
you want to be.

My Darkest Desire

Sometimes it's hard to admit what we really want sexually, even to ourselves. Let's take a moment to dig deep and find out what your darkest, most depraved desire really is.

Are you unsure whether you even have a dark desire? Think back to dreams that made you blush when you thought about them the next day, or fleeting thoughts you might have had when your boss comes into your office. Having a dark desire is not unusual. You're not alone. You can prove this simply by doing a quick Internet search on the desire that came to your mind; chances are you'll find a forum with people questioning their own penchant for silk ties and goggles. Don't judge yourself for having these kinky thoughts, but, at the same time don't act on a thought unless it's safe, sane, and consensual.

TO TAP INTO your darkest desire, you have to let go of your inhibitions first. Turn the lights off, light a candle, and play some music that turns you on. Now make sure that you are alone, behind locked doors. Start by writing the following phrase:

> "I will not judge my darkest desire. When I'm all alone and fantasizing about sex, what I really want is
>
> _____
>
> _____
>
> _____ ."

Fill in the blank with the first thing that comes to mind. I'm not going to give you any specific ideas here. Let it come naturally and be truly what you want.

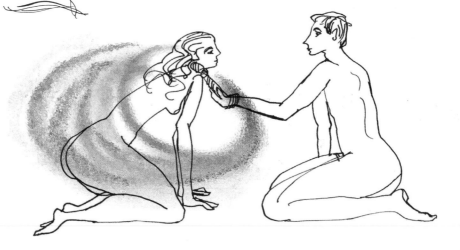

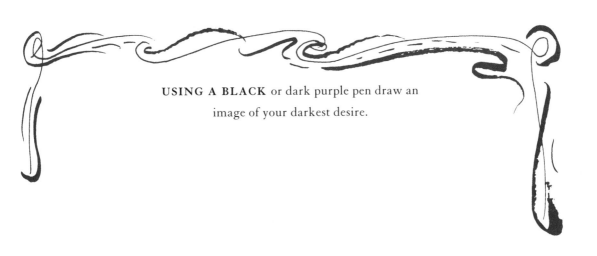

USING A BLACK or dark purple pen draw an
image of your darkest desire.

"Those who restrain desire do so because theirs is weak enough to be restrained."
—WILLIAM BLAKE, *THE MARRIAGE OF HEAVEN AND HELL*

Dirty Dreams

Have you ever had a dirty dream? I mean a *really* dirty dream, one where you woke up aroused and thought about it for days? One where you blushed when you saw the object of your dreamtime affection? Use these pages to explore the naughty side of your subconscious.

Do you have a particularly kinky desire that you'd love for your partner to fulfill, but you're not sure what his or her reaction will be (e.g., a threesome or a bondage experience)? To gauge your partner's reaction to your idea, try framing your desire as if it were only a dream. For example, say, "Honey, I had the strangest dream last night about us having a threesome with our neighbor!" If he is excited by your naughty dream, then start a conversation about it—and if the conversation goes well, perhaps suggest that you two could make your dream a reality someday! If, on the other hand, he is disinterested or disturbed by your idea, you can always chalk it up to being only a dream.

RECALL A SEXY dream that you've had about someone and record it in as much detail as possible here. Who were you with? Was it someone you knew? Or a made-up entity? Was it someone who you would sleep with in real life? What were the circumstances of your encounter? Did anything really unusual or provocative occur? Would you want any of this dream to come true in real life? Why or why not?

_____

_____

_____

_____

_____

_____

_____

_____

_____

_____

_____

_____

_____

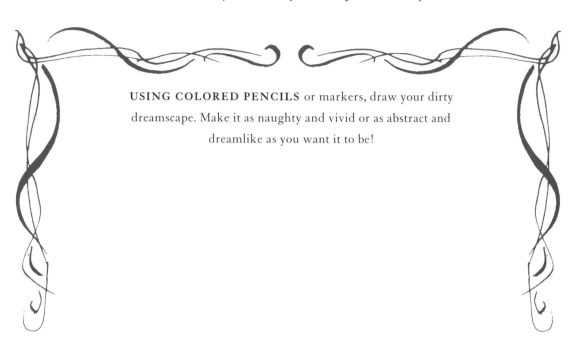

"I'll let you be in my dreams if I can be in yours." —BOB DYLAN

USING COLORED PENCILS or markers, draw your dirty
dreamscape. Make it as naughty and vivid or as abstract and
dreamlike as you want it to be!

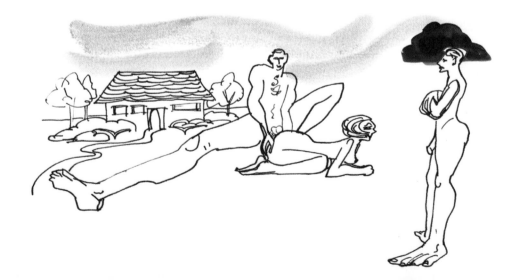

The Most Romantic Gesture

What is the most romantic gesture your partner could ever give you? Use these pages to explore what romance means to you. You may find that your idea of romance is not what you thought it would be!

WRITE DOWN ten romantic gestures that you would like for your current or potential partner to share with you to show you that he or she really cares. They can be sexy, romantic, or even practical—just make sure they are actions that would really make you feel loved.

"It would be romantic if . . ."

_____

_____

_____

_____

_____

_____

_____

_____

_____

_____

_____

_____

_____

_____

_____

_____

_____

_____

Often we get comfortable with our partners and forget to show them that we are still crazy about them. Take those ten romantic gestures that you wrote down and put them on little slips of paper and toss them in a hat or a shoebox. Ask your lover to do the same. Choose a day of the week, perhaps Monday, or a day of the month, such as the first, to pull a slip of paper out of the box. The goal is to have one partner fulfill the romantic gesture for the other before the end of the week or month!

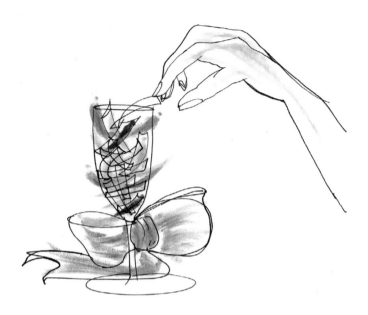

WRITE A MESSAGE IN A BOTTLE. You'll need a glass bottle (ideally one with a cork in it—a clear wine bottle left over from a romantic date works great), stickers to decorate the bottle, a pretty piece of stationery, (optional) a sexy photo of yourself, a ribbon, and confetti.

WRITE A SEXY or romantic message on the stationery; you can address it to yourself (to open at a later date) or to your lover. Include a sexy photo of yourself, if you like, and roll the message and photo together and tie it with a ribbon. Drop the message into the bottle and sprinkle in some confetti. Cork the bottle. Decorate the outside as you like with stickers or anything other flourishes that suit you, and tie a ribbon around the neck. Give it to your lover as a romantic gift, or give it to yourself to open at a later date when you need a self-esteem boost.

> *"And he took her in his arms and kissed her under the sunlit sky, and he cared not that they stood high upon the walls in the sight of many."* —J.R.R. TOLKIEN, *RETURN OF THE KING*

My Heart Belongs To . . .

Who does your heart really belong to?
What person makes your heart swell
and overflow with feelings of love and
desire? Use these pages to explore who
makes your heart go *boom boom boom*.

Expressing love for your
romantic partner during sex
can improve the experience
and reaffirm your intimate
connection. The next time
you are in the throes of
passion, take a second to lock
eyes with your partner and
whisper, "I love you."
In a truly loving relationship,
this moment of vulnerable
intimacy can open the
floodgates of passion
and heighten the sexual
experience.

WHEN YOU THINK about romantic love, who comes to mind? Write down who holds the keys to your heart. Is it locked up in the hands of your lover? Do you still pine for a long-lost love? Does your heart belong to no one but yourself? Describe how you know that you love this person, or describe why you don't love anyone. (Are you afraid? Have you just not found the right person?) Really dig into what it means to you to be in love.

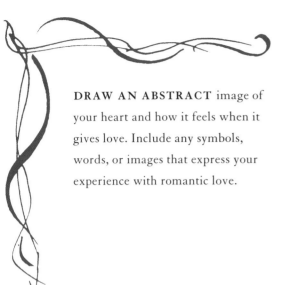

DRAW AN ABSTRACT image of your heart and how it feels when it gives love. Include any symbols, words, or images that express your experience with romantic love.

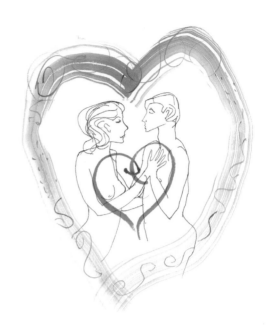

"I love you without knowing how, or when, or from where. I love you simply, without problems or pride: I love you in this way because I do not know any other way of loving but this, in which there is no I or you, so intimate that your hand upon my chest is my hand, so intimate that when I fall asleep your eyes close." —PABLO NERUDA, *100 LOVE SONNETS*

My Perfect Sexperience

Have you ever experienced
a sexual encounter that
was just absolutely *perfect*?
Use these pages to uncover
the ingredients of your
most blissful sexperience.

THINK BACK TO a sexual
encounter (or encounters)
that left your toes tingling
and knees quaking—the type
of experience that you
couldn't stop replaying in
your mind the next day while
making copies at work, the
type of experience that you
still think about while masturbating. What made this
experience stand out? Who
was there? What happened?
Have you ever felt anything
like it again? If not, why not?
Is there any way to have this
type of experience again?

> *"Sex without love is a meaningless experience, but as far as meaningless experiences go it's pretty damn good."*
> —WOODY ALLEN, AMERICAN WRITER AND DIRECTOR

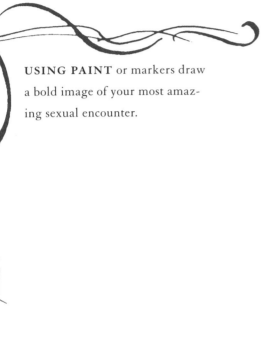

USING PAINT or markers draw a bold image of your most amazing sexual encounter.

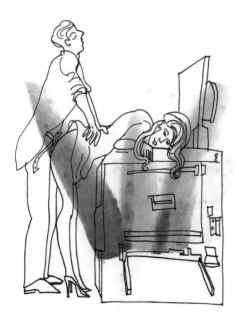

How I Really Feel About Intimacy

Intimacy with a lover can often be confused with sex. But true intimacy is about being emotionally vulnerable with a partner, which can improve the quality of your shared sex life. Use these pages to explore how you really feel about intimacy.

ANSWER THE FOLLOWING questions to get yourself thinking about your experiences with intimacy.

In my life, with which romantic partner have I felt most intimate?

_____

Do I share emotional intimacy with my current partner?

_____

_____

What is the most intimate (emotionally and sexually vulnerable) experience I've ever shared with a partner?

_____

_____

_____

_____

Do I enjoy kissing and hugging my current partner?

_____

_____

Do I need intimacy to enjoy sex? Why, or why not?

_____

_____

_____

_____

_____

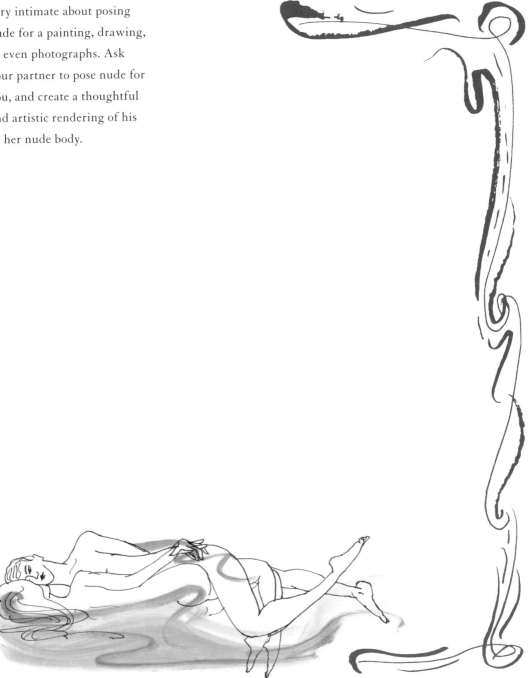

"Among men, sex sometimes results in intimacy;
among women, intimacy sometimes results in sex."
—BARBARA CARTLAND, ENGLISH AUTHOR

THERE IS SOMETHING

very intimate about posing
nude for a painting, drawing,
or even photographs. Ask
your partner to pose nude for
you, and create a thoughtful
and artistic rendering of his
or her nude body.

What Arousal Feels Like

How do you know
when you're aroused?
Use these pages to
express what being
horny feels like to you.

TO EXPLORE YOUR AROUSAL, start by thinking about the following questions: Do you feel a tingling or aching sensation in your lower abdomen, your thighs, or your toes? Without touching yourself can you tell if you are wet? How do you normally respond to your arousal? Do you instigate sex with your partner? Do you masturbate? Do you ignore it? Is feeling horny a welcome and wanted sensation for you?

Describe in detail how it feels to be turned on.

_____

_____

_____

_____

_____

_____

_____

"There are a number of mechanical devices which increase sexual arousal, particularly in women. Chief among these is the Mercedes-Benz 380SL convertible."
—P. J. O'ROURKE, AMERICAN POLITICAL SATIRIST

Think about the times that you've been most aroused in your life. What exactly were the elements that got you there? Write a list of the top ten turn-ons and see if you can find a theme. Once you've articulated your turn-ons, then you can make an effort to seek out those experiences and consciously amp up your sex life.

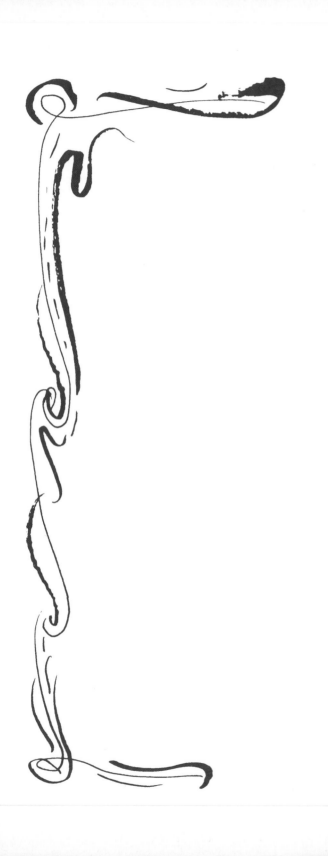

THE NEXT TIME you enjoy a sexual experience, whether alone or with a partner, try to visualize it as a trek through the mountains. You may start out wandering through a field of pleasure slowly breathing in the sweet scents, and then you begin a hike up a steep hill of arousal, your heartbeat increases, your breathing quickens . . . Afterward, draw your mountainous journey using a vibrant set of pastels; record the fields, peaks, and valleys that you encounter and see where your journey takes you.

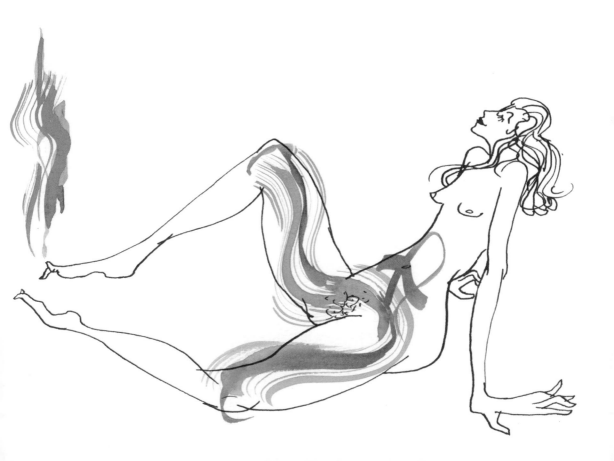

I Like To Be Touched . . .

So much of the sexual experience is about touching and being touched. We often narrow our focus to simply touching the genitals. But what happens when your lover touches the inside of your wrist with the tips of his fingers? The small of your back with the flat expanse of his palm? What if he uses his lips to touch the nape of your neck? Do these touches send frissons down your legs, a jolt of pleasure to your core?

WRITE DOWN ten different ways that you enjoy being touched. Describe in detail how exactly this type of touch makes your body respond. Here's an example: "When my lover traces his tongue up the inside of my thigh, my whole body tenses in anticipation, and I see colors."

Let's explore the realm of touch and create an erogenous map of your body. Have your lover blindfold you, and lie fully naked on a comfortable surface, arms relaxed by your side. Allow your lover to explore your body with his hands, starting from the crown of your head, moving along your face, your neck, shoulders, arms, hands, chest, stomach, thighs, shins, and feet. Turn over and let him explore your back. As he lingers in each region, let him know whether he's found a sensitive spot by giving a verbal rating on this scale:

~

Saying ONE means you don't like it when he touches that spot.

~

Saying TWO means you feel neutral about him touching that spot.

~

Saying THREE means you like it when he touches that spot.

~

Saying FOUR means it turns you on when he touches that spot.

~

Saying FIVE means that touching that spot could lead to orgasm.

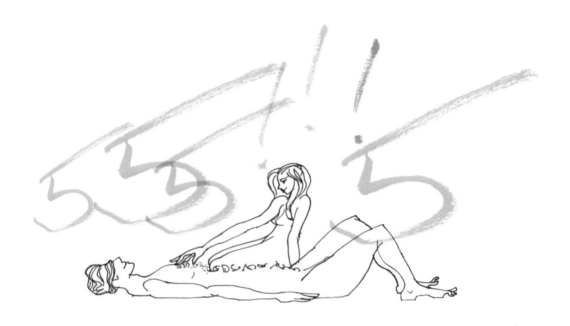

DRAW YOUR PERSONAL erogenous map. Start with a photo or drawing of yourself standing, full length (nude would be best), then color in each spot on your body in a shade that shows how sensitive you are. The color red could indicate an orgasmic zone, purple could indicate a part of your body that you find relaxing to be caressed, and gray could indicate a spot where you don't like to be touched at all.

"See how she leans her cheek upon her hand. / O that I were a glove upon that hand / That I might touch that cheek!"
—WILLIAM SHAKESPEARE, *ROMEO AND JULIET*

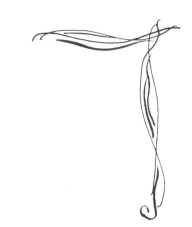

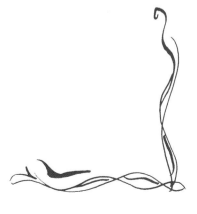

On Orgasms

Every woman's orgasm is a little bit different, and even one woman can have orgasms that are as varied as the colors in a box of crayons. Use these pages to explore the beauty of your unique orgasmic experience.

MY ORGASM FEELS LIKE . . .

_____

_____

_____

_____

_____

_____

_____

_____

_____

_____

_____

_____

Do you have difficulty achieving orgasm during sex? You're not alone, according to Brown University, one in three women can't find the big O they're looking for. Common inhibitors include shyness with a partner or a partner that doesn't quite know how to touch you. The first step to achieving orgasm during partnered sex is to learn how to climax solo. Explore your body using your fingers or a sex toy to discover the right pressure, stroke, and fantasy that puts you over the top. Once you've mastered solo pleasure, share the information you've learned about yourself with your partner. Don't be shy; you're already naked with this guy, so you may as well let your inhibitions fly.

"Electric flesh-arrows . . . traversing the body. A rainbow of color strikes the eyelids. A foam of music falls over the ears. It is the gong of the orgasm." —ANAÏS NIN

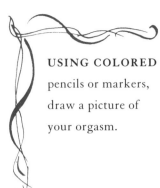

USING COLORED
pencils or markers,
draw a picture of
your orgasm.

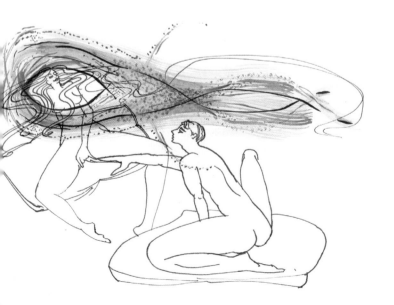

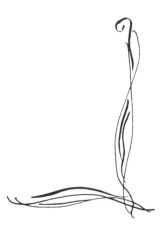

The Taste of Sex

Great sex touches all five of your senses, not the least of which is your sense of taste. Use these pages to explore how your sense of taste ignites during sex.

WHAT DOES SEX with your partner *taste* like? Salty, pungent, earthy, strong, raw? These are a few words that may come to mind. Think about how it tastes when you put your tongue to your partner's sex. Can you describe in full detail the taste of his cum? What about the taste of her kiss? Write down at least ten adjectives that accurately describe the flavors of sex. If you are having trouble coming up with adjectives, try to compare it to foods that you've tasted. (Oysters, anyone?)

_____

_____

_____

_____

_____

_____

_____

_____

_____

_____

_____

_____

"Clinton lied. A man might forget where he parks or where he lives, but he never forgets oral sex, no matter how bad it is."
—BARBARA BUSH, FORMER U.S. FIRST LADY

Have you ever swallowed your partner's cum? There's something to be said about a woman who goes the extra mile and relishes in the flavor of her lover's juices. If you haven't taken that leap of taste, try the following to make sure it goes down smoothly:

~

Shoot it like a tequila shot! The second your partner squirts in your mouth, push his penis to the back of your throat, past the taste buds, and swallow it down.

~

Dress it up! Add flavored lube, whipped cream, or chocolate sauce, whatever it takes to make the flavor more palatable to you.

~

Enjoy it! There is something very intimate about taking your lover's juices into your mouth. Think about how naughty you feel and how aroused it makes you (and your partner!), and you may just find that you really love the stuff. You'll never know if you don't try!

~

Try it in the morning. Your gag reflex is less responsive in the morning, and it's easier to swallow your lover's cum on an empty stomach.

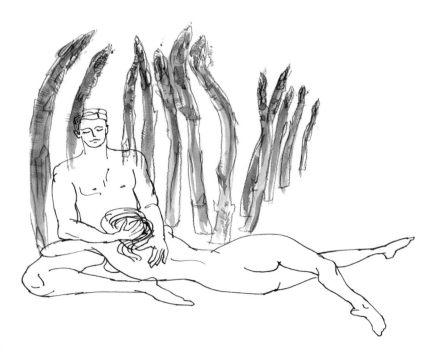

Blindfolded

By taking away your sense of sight, you'll be able to focus on the other sensations that envelop your body during a sexual experience. Use these pages to explore the appeal of using a blindfold during sex play.

Play the sexy version of the "What is it?" game. Blindfold your partner and introduce some sexy surprises into the bedroom to tickle his or her senses:

~

Food items such as whipped cream, strawberries, and honey. Have your partner taste these items and guess what they are, and then drizzle some on his or her naked body—and lick them off.

Sex toys such as dildos, handcuffs, nipple clamps, and vibrators. Use these items on your partner's body and ask him or her to describe how it feels when you use them.

Sensation items such as feather ticklers, spanking paddles, ice cubes, and body candle wax. Surprise your partner's senses with these extreme sensations and ask your partner to describe what he or she is feeling.

PLAY THE ROLE of the blindfolded partner as described in the sex tip exercise on this page. After playtime is over, write down how the sensations felt on your body and how being blindfolded contributed to the experience. Or play the leading role and ask your partner to describe his or her sensations as you deliver them. Write everything down. You may find you have the material needed to put together a vivid and sexy poem. Give it a try!

GET CREATIVE AND try some blindfolded body painting. For this project you'll need a sheet, a blindfold, body paint, a willing partner or yourself. Spread a sheet over the ground to protect your flooring from paint spills. Have your partner blindfold you. Now paint the skin of your nude partner by first dipping your hands and fingers in the body paint and then running your hands over the contours of your partner's body. When you feel like you've covered most of your partner's skin, remove your blindfold and see the masterpiece you've created.

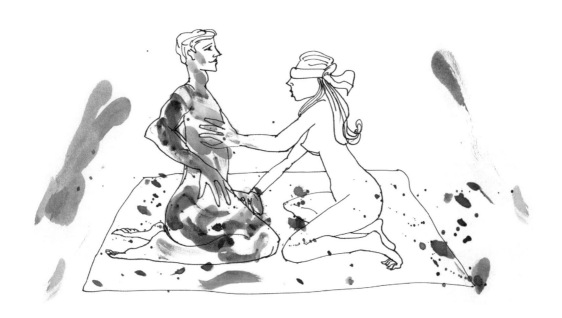

"Who can blind lover's eyes?" — VIRGIL, ANCIENT ROMAN POET

I Feel Sexiest When . . .

To truly have a fulfilling sex life, it's
important to pay attention to what
makes you feel sexy. Use these pages to
explore your sexy side.

Feeling sexy is a state of mind. Here are some easy steps
to being as sexy as you wanna be:

~

**Take a pole-dancing, striptease, or belly-dancing class at your local
dance studio.** Learning to feel comfortable in your own skin is the best
way to feel sexy.

~

Self-care. Get your nails done (or do them yourself). Invest in some
daring, red lipstick. Visit a salon and enjoy a massage and a makeover.
By taking the time to take care of yourself, you are giving yourself
permission to feel sexy.

~

Sex up your alone time. Read erotica while taking a hot bath. Toss
your husband's T-shirt in the hamper and sleep in a sexy silk nightie
for a change. Just add one extra, little sexy activity to your normal
routine and see how it makes you feel.

"What a thing of fantasy a woman may become after dusk."
—HONORE DE BALZAC, *FERRAGUS, CHEF DES DÉVORANTS*

WRITE DOWN THE TOP TEN things that make you feel sexy. Start with "I feel sexiest when . . ." and fill in the blanks.

LOOK AT YOURSELF in the mirror. What is your sexiest feature? Is it your eyes? Your breasts? The length of your thighs? Using a pencil, draw this feature in detail. Instead of using shading strokes with your pencil, write *sexy, sexy, sexy* over and over to create the shaded parts.

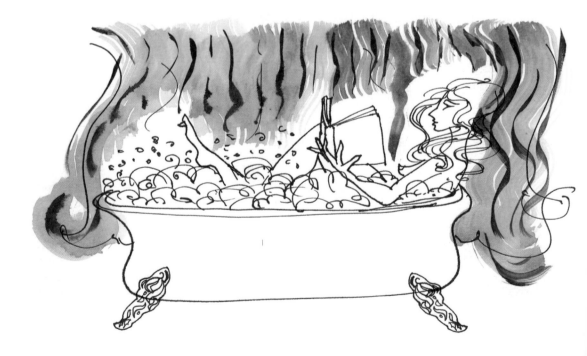

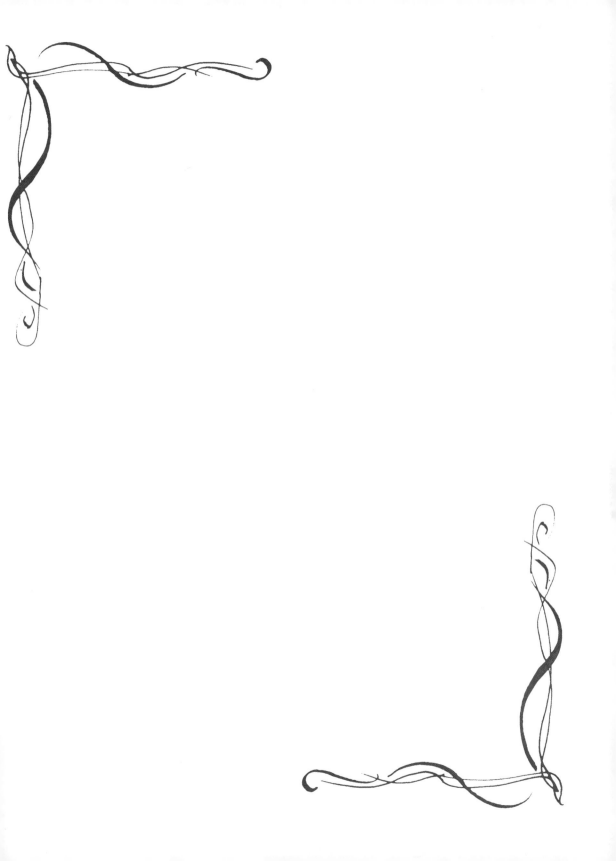

Vulva Map

If you spread your legs and look between your thighs, all the beautiful, tender parts that you see are part of your vulva. We often don't take the time to really look at and admire it in all its feminine power. Use these pages to discover the unique beauty of your own pleasure center.

Your clitoris is actually an organ that is made up of eighteen different parts (including the labia, clitoral shaft, crura/legs, and G-spot, among others) and contains a whopping 8,000 nerve endings. In fact, it is said to measure up to eight full inches when regarded as a complete organ.

LET'S UNCOVER HOW YOU FEEL about your sexy parts. Answer the following questions:

Do you think your vulva is pretty or ugly? Why?

_____

What color is your vulva? _____

Do you think that your vulva should look like everyone else's? Why? _____

_____

Is your clitoral bulb (the nub of your clitoris) big or small? Is it exposed, or hidden behind a hood?

_____

Are your inner labia (lips) symmetrical? Are they long? Are they short? Describe them in detail.

_____

Do you keep your pubic hair trimmed or shaved, or do you let it run wild? What color is your hair down there? Do you have intimate piercings or tattoos, or do you vajazzle (decorate with crystals)?

_____

What do you like about your vulva, clitoris, or vagina?

_____

Describe the scent of your sexual secretions. Do you like the way they smell?

_____

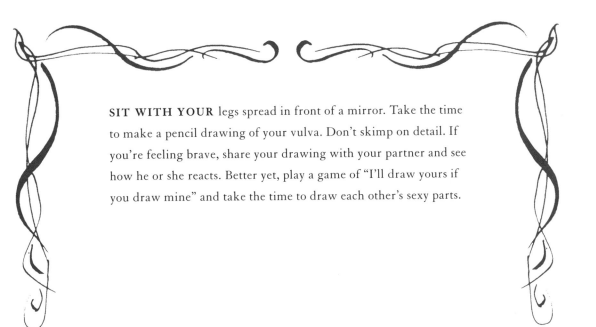

SIT WITH YOUR legs spread in front of a mirror. Take the time to make a pencil drawing of your vulva. Don't skimp on detail. If you're feeling brave, share your drawing with your partner and see how he or she reacts. Better yet, play a game of "I'll draw yours if you draw mine" and take the time to draw each other's sexy parts.

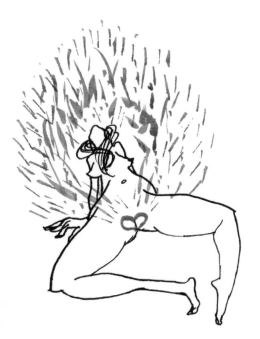

"[The clitoris has] . . . a higher concentration of nerve fibers than is found anywhere else on the body, including the fingertips, lips, and tongue, and it is twice the number in the penis. In a sense, then, a woman's little brain is bigger than a man's." —NATALIE ANGIER, *WOMAN: AN INTIMATE GEOGRAPHY*

My Body, My Best

When you love and accept your body as it is and yourself exactly as you are, your sex life will improve dramatically. Use these pages to explore the things you love most about your body and yourself.

WRITE DOWN one hundred things that you love about your body (e.g., your adorable toes!), yourself (e.g., your outgoing personality!), and your sexuality (e.g., you give amazing head!). By not stopping until you uncover one hundred wonderful things about yourself, you'll be able to move past some of the more superficial things you love and really dig deep into what makes you beautifully unique. Keep this list handy for whenever you feel low on self-esteem.

_____ _____ _____ _____

_____ _____ _____ _____

_____ _____ _____ _____

_____ _____ _____ _____

_____ _____ _____ _____

_____ _____ _____ _____

_____ _____ _____ _____

_____ _____ _____ _____

_____ _____ _____ _____

_____ _____ _____ _____

_____ _____ _____ _____

_____ _____ _____ _____

_____ _____ _____ _____

_____ _____ _____ _____

_____ _____ _____ _____

_____ _____ _____ _____

_____ _____ _____ _____

_____ _____ _____ _____

_____ _____ _____ _____

_____ _____ _____ _____

HAVE SOMEONE take a photo of your fully nude body. Now take a printout of this photo and use it to draw a self-portrait using pencil or charcoal. Treat the image as if it is one of a stranger and try to really appreciate all the beautiful aspects of this person that you are drawing.

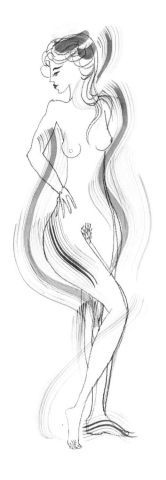

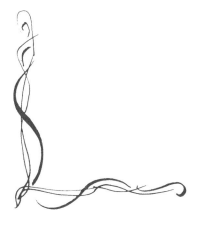

"She wins who calls herself beautiful and challenges the world to change to truly see her."
—NAOMI WOLF, *THE BEAUTY MYTH: HOW IMAGES OF BEAUTY ARE USED AGAINST WOMEN*

Masturbation

Masturbation is an integral part of your sex life. Use these pages to express your thoughts on self-pleasure.

WRITE DOWN THE STORY of your typical masturbation session. What do you do to consistently bring yourself to orgasm? Do you use a sex toy or your fingers? Do you masturbate in bed? The shower? Your office? How often do you self-pleasure? Who or what do you fantasize about? Do you watch porn? If so, what type? Do you completely undress? Do you wear lingerie?

Review your masturbation story from time to time (as you've written it on this page). If you check back in a year or so and discover that you are still doing the same ol' thing, it's time to try something fun and new! For example, if you don't usually watch porn, add some porn into your solo time. If you always play with yourself in bed, try the shower. Masturbation is a part of your sex life, and just like with partnered sex, you don't want to get stuck in a rut, so make an effort to change things up.

_____

_____

_____

_____

_____

_____

_____

_____

_____

_____

_____

_____

_____

_____

MAKE A SELF-PLEASURE video. Using the camera on your laptop or your cell phone take a video (not including your face) of your masturbation session. As you review the video, pause it on a frame that you find particularly sexy and draw or paint a reproduction of it!

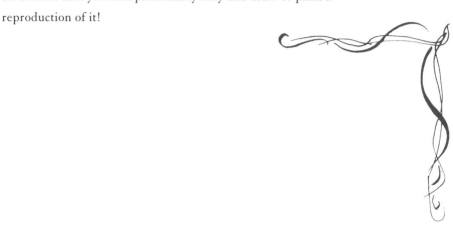

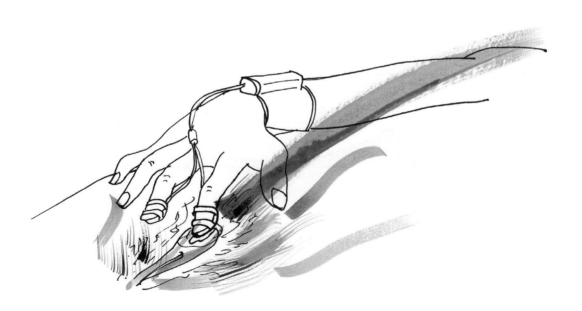

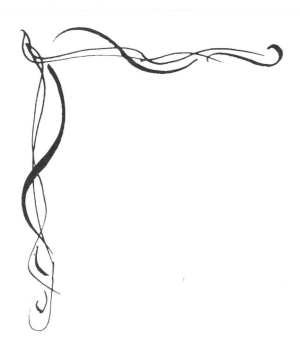

"The good thing about masturbation is that you don't have to get dressed up for it."
—TRUMAN CAPOTE, AMERICAN AUTHOR

My O Face

When you orgasm, you probably exhibit a unique facial expression that pop culture has dubbed the O face (orgasm face). Use these pages to get to know and appreciate your O face.

HAVE YOU EVER considered your O face? What does it look like? Try having sex or masturbating in front of a mirror and focusing on your face at times of extreme pleasure, or ask your partner to help describe what your expressions of sexual pleasure might look like. Come up with a complete sentence or paragraph about your orgasmic expression.

"If things go well I might be showing her my O face. 'Oh . . . Oh . . . Oh!' You know what I'm talkin' about. 'Oh!'" —DREW FROM THE FILM *OFFICE SPACE*

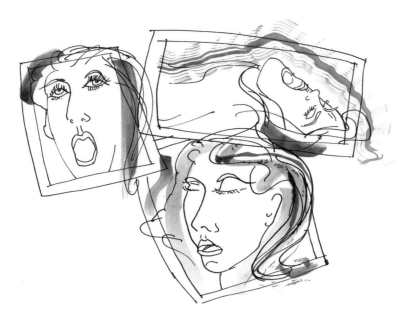

HAVE YOUR PARTNER take a photograph of your face—just your face—at the moment of orgasm. Create a collection of these photos and turn them into a collage or a scrapbook. You may also choose to begin collecting and collaging photos of your lovers' faces as they approach orgasm (with their consent, of course).

According to relationship expert and author Tracey Cox, men, in particular, love watching your face during sex. She says, "Most men—justifiably—believe our facial expression provides the best possible indicator of whether or not we're faking orgasm." To truly enjoy sex, it's important for you to let go of your inhibitions and let your partner see the pleasure that he's providing.

My Partner's Body

How do you feel about your partner's body? Does it arouse you? Make you feel safe? Does it make you feel warm and loved? Use these pages to explore your relationship with your partner's (or partners'!) body.

WRITE DOWN AT LEAST TWENTY reasons you love your partner's body. What are your favorite parts of his or her body? How does your partner's body make you feel? If you don't have a partner at the moment, think back to previous partners or think about your current crush or idealized lover.

Your partner loves hearing compliments! Make a concerted effort this week to give him at least one or two compliments about his physical body every single day. They can be as sweet (e.g., "I love how safe I feel wrapped in your big arms") or as sexy (e.g., "You have the most amazing cock!") as you want them to be. Making your partner feel good about himself will make you feel good too!

"The body is meant to be seen, not all covered up."
—MARILYN MONROE, AMERICAN ACTRESS

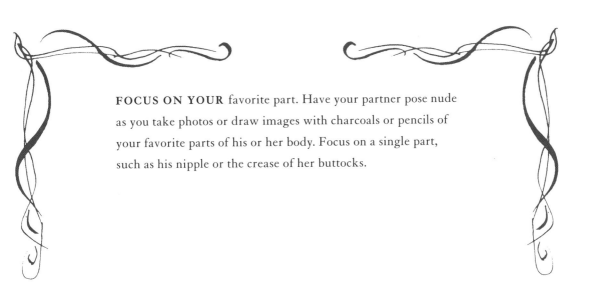

FOCUS ON YOUR favorite part. Have your partner pose nude as you take photos or draw images with charcoals or pencils of your favorite parts of his or her body. Focus on a single part, such as his nipple or the crease of her buttocks.

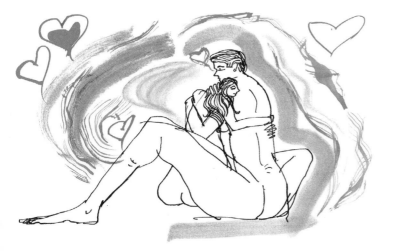

My Crushes

Whether you're in a relationship or not, you probably harbor a secret (or not-so-secret) crush on someone. Use these pages to explore the people who you find sexiest and most arousing in this world.

The euphoric feeling of a full-blown crush is largely related to chemical factors in our brains. If your crush makes you feel giddy, you're probably under the influence of dopamine. This naturally occurring chemical neurotransmitter releases in your brain whenever anything good happens, including when you get an eyeful of Mr. McDreamy from the seventh floor. Other things that can cause dopamine release are eating chocolate and exercise.

WRITE DOWN A detailed description of your crush, without revealing his or her name. Express what you'd like to experience with your crush: Are you interested in a sexual tryst? Do you have a relationship fantasy? Other questions to ponder: Is there any chance that your dreams with this person will ever come true? Does your crush know you exist? Do you want him or her to?

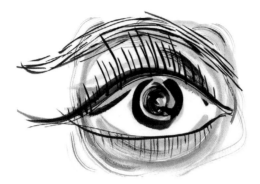
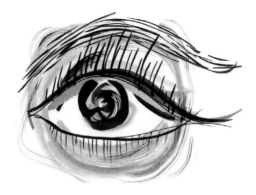

DRAW A SKETCH of your crush, emphasize the attributes that particularly excite you. For example, if he has amazing eyes, draw his image in black and white but give his eyes a burst of color.

Thinking about Penis

Penises are peculiar things, aren't they? They are simultaneously soft (to the touch) and hard (when erect). They are funny looking, yet can be so provocative and exciting in the right context. Use these pages to investigate your feelings for the penis.

WRITE IN AS MUCH DETAIL as possible how you feel about penis. Here are some questions to get you started: What is your perfect size? Do you like them with a particular bend? Have you ever had a partner in your life who you considered to have "the perfect penis"? What made it perfect to you? How do you feel about the way penises look? The way they feel? How many penises have you encountered in your lifetime?

_____

_____

_____

_____

_____

_____

_____

_____

_____

_____

_____

_____

_____

_____

It's difficult not to please the penis, the male's pleasure center. Take note that the majority of men report that the most sensitive spot (in a good way) is their frenulum. This is the little strip of flesh on the underside of his shaft that connects the shaft to head. Gently caress this spot with your thumb or lick it with the tip of your tongue during oral sex.

"See, the problem is that God gives men a brain and a penis, and only enough blood to run one at a time." —ROBIN WILLIAMS

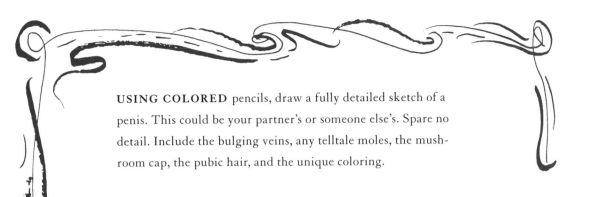

USING COLORED pencils, draw a fully detailed sketch of a penis. This could be your partner's or someone else's. Spare no detail. Include the bulging veins, any telltale moles, the mushroom cap, the pubic hair, and the unique coloring.

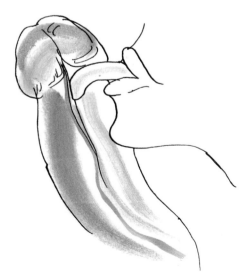

Switching Sides

Have you ever switched sides and had sex with a partner of the opposite gender than you are typically attracted to? Use these pages to explore how this made—or would make—you feel.

DESCRIBE YOUR EXPERIENCE in detail with exploring alternative sexual orientations. Who did you explore with? What were the circumstances of your encounter? Was it exciting? Disappointing? Was it worth repeating? If you've never experienced this, would you want to? Do you have any secret fantasies about exploring sex outside of your sexual orientation? Why or why not?

"I like pin-up girls. I'm more of a boy than a girl. I'm not a lesbian, though—not before a sambuca anyway." —AMY WINEHOUSE, ENGLISH SINGER-SONGWRITER

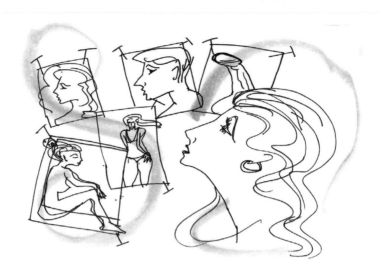

"Cut the ending. Revise the script. The man of her dreams is a girl." —JULIE ANNE PETERS, *KEEPING YOU A SECRET*

MAKE A COLLAGE of people (famous or not) that you find attractive who do not represent your typical sexual orientation. Do you notice anything in common among them?

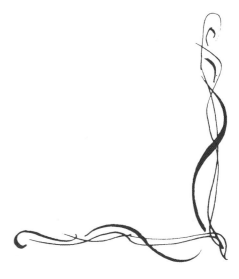

I Am an Exhibitionist

Do you like the idea of being watched while having sex, undressing, or masturbating? Does it give you a thrill to put on a show? Use these pages to explore your exhibitionist side.

Engaging in exhibitionism doesn't necessarily mean that you need to let go of all feelings of shyness or insecurity. In fact, it's this feeling of vulnerability that makes exhibitionism that much more fun and thrilling! If you find yourself playing a bit of the coquette while giving your voyeuristic partner a show, know that you are perfectly playing the part of the sexual exhibitionist.

DESCRIBE ANY MEMORABLE exhibitionist experiences you've had or any exhibitionistic fantasies you harbor. Here are some questions to get you started: Have you ever had sex where someone could watch you—maybe at a party or at a swinger's club? Have you ever purposefully left your window shades open and your lights on while undressing? Are you excited by the idea of being observed while engaging in a sexual act? Would you describe yourself as an exhibitionist? Why or why not?

HAVE YOUR partner take photos of you as you undress, masturbate, or engage in a sexual act in front of him or her.

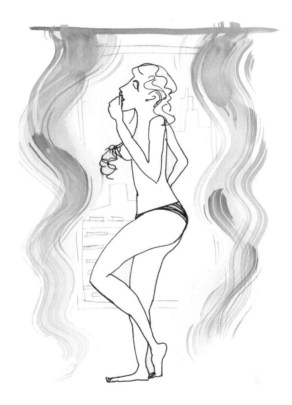

"I won't be satisfied until people want to hear me sing without looking at me. Of course, that doesn't mean I want them to stop looking." —MARILYN MONROE

I Am a Voyeur

Do you like to watch other people engage in sexual acts in front of you? Are you content to sit on the sidelines and enjoy the show? Use these pages to explore your voyeuristic side.

WRITE DOWN YOUR EXPERIENCE with voyeurism. Here are some questions to get you started: Have you ever secretly watched someone else having sex? Perhaps through a bedroom window when your neighbor in the building across the way left the lights on and curtains open? Have you ever watched someone having sex in person, maybe at a club or a party? Does the idea of watching your partner have sex with someone else excite you? How does it make you feel to sit on the sidelines and watch other people in the throes of passion? Would you consider yourself to be a voyeur? Why or why not?

When exploring voyeurism, as in all things sexual, make sure that your activities are safe, sane, and consensual. Many states have "peeping tom" laws, and if you engage in nonconsensual voyeurism you could find yourself on the wrong side of the law. The moral of the story is it's okay to be a voyeur, but make sure that you aren't violating anyone else's privacy in the act.

_____

_____

_____

_____

_____

_____

_____

_____

_____

_____

_____

_____

_____

_____

_____

_____

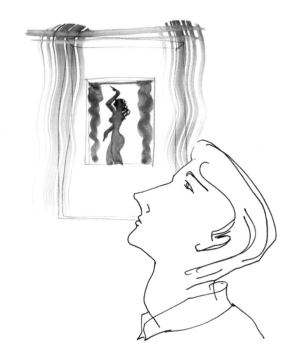

> *"The exhibitionist is nothing*
> *without the voyeur, and vice-a-versa."*
> —JONATHAN LIGHT, *THE ART OF PORN*

WITH A WILLING partner, take photos or a video of him or her while he or she is engaged in a sexual act, whether that be masturbating, undressing, or having sex with someone else.

Daring Locations I Want To Try

Sex shouldn't just be about getting it on in the bedroom. It can be so much fun to enjoy a sexy encounter in a place that's just a bit more adventurous. Use these pages to explore the daring locations you want to try.

There is an art to having sex in a daring location. Choose a location that feels dangerous but where your actual odds of getting discovered are slim—for example, off a hiking trail in the woods, or in a public restroom that has only one toilet rather than stalls. Wear clothing that is easy to take off and on. The last thing you want is to struggle putting your clothes back on in the event that you need to quickly dress. Having an encounter during the nighttime is safer than during the daytime because the darkness affords more privacy, no matter where you are.

LIST AT LEAST TWENTY places outside of the bedroom where you want to experience a sexual encounter. Be creative! Here are a few ideas to get you started: in a ski gondola, in a public restroom, at a night club . . .

_____

_____

_____

_____

_____

_____

_____

_____

_____

_____

_____

_____

CREATE A SEXY MAP. Make a collage of all the daring locations that you want to try by cutting and pasting images from magazines or printouts from the Web. Hang the map on your bedroom wall. Each time you and your lover enjoy a daring romp together, put a pin in the map. See if you can travel the entirety of your sexy map.

"Sex is the most fun you can have without laughing." —WOODY ALLEN

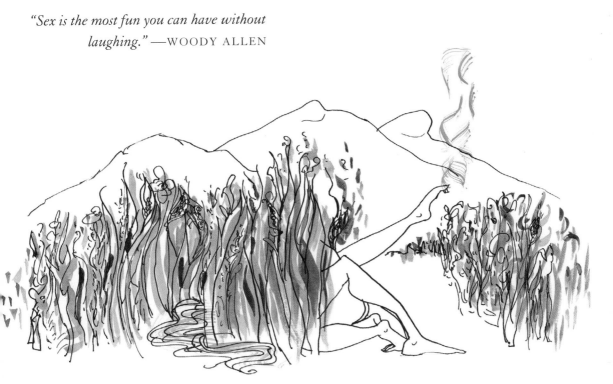

Back-Door Adventures

To some women, anal sex is an integral and exciting part of the sexual experience; for others, it's unchartered territory. Use these pages to explore your experience with, and feelings about, back-door adventures.

The anus does not produce its own lubrication, so be sure to stock up on some slippery stuff before you go to "fifth base." You can use water-based or oil-based lubes for anal sex, but if you plan to double your lube and use it for vaginal intercourse, then select a water-based lube. The more natural the better. Another thing to remember is, if you want to pursue anal sex, it's important to keep everything clean back there and make sure your penetrating partner wraps it up with a condom.

WRITE DOWN YOUR feelings about exploring anal. Have you ever had anal sex? Why or why not? If you haven't, are you willing to try? Why or why not? If you have, how was your experience? Have you ever experienced an orgasm during anal sex?

_____

_____

_____

_____

_____

_____

_____

_____

_____

_____

"Let me make it very clear . . . Any man I contemplate has to be into anal sex . . . Yes, I 'do anal' and in fact I would be deeply unhappy if 'doing anal' wasn't on the menu . . ."
—SINEAD O'CONNOR, IRISH SINGER-SONGWRITER

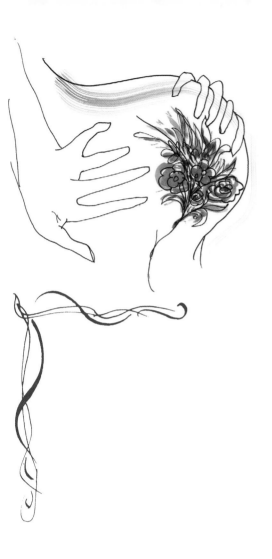

DRAW AN IMAGE OF YOUR ANUS.
You can make it a very literal interpretation and even use a hand mirror to do a precise portrait, or you can make it an abstract interpretation (e.g., hidden doorways or a secret garden). This exercise is intended to remind you to feel comfortable with all aspects of your body. It's all you!

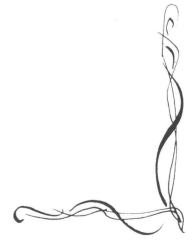

I Am Dominant . . .

Strap on your stilettos
and grab your whip:
It's time to explore
your dominant side.
Use these pages to
tap into your inner
(or outer!) dominatrix.

WRITE IN DETAIL about your experience with domination.
Here are some questions to get you started: Have you ever
dominated during sex? If yes, how did it feel? If no, why not?
Describe in detail a sexy scenario (real or imagined) where
you've played the role of the dominant partner. If you've never
dominated, is this something you'd like to try? If so, what's
stopping you?

Dominating in bed doesn't
necessarily require you to
wear a leather catsuit and
handle a whip. Sometimes
it's just a matter of taking
initiative and calling the
shots. Call all the shots for at
least one intimate session.
This means *you* decide when
it's time for sex, *you* decide
what position you want, and
you demand the oral sex (or
whatever you desire!). You
may find it to be a
very empowering and
exciting experience.

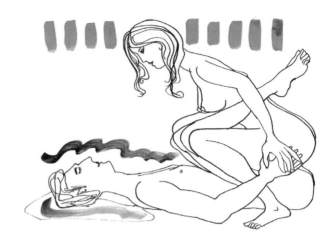

USING MARKERS, DRAW an image of what being sexually dominating means to you. You can make it as realistic or as abstract/symbolic as you like.

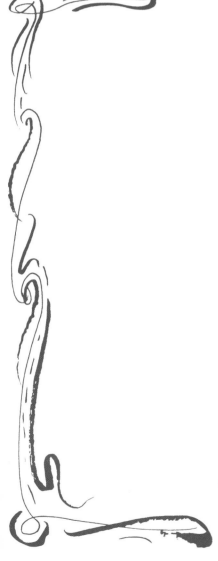

"How do you decide you wanna be a dominatrix? What, do you wake up one day and go, 'Hey, I feel like being bossy'?"
—SHEILA KINGSTON, *EXIT TO EDEN*

I Am Submissive . . .

Surrender to submission. Use these pages to explore your submissive tendencies.

As women in the twenty-first century, we wear many hats during a day and take on endless responsibilities. This makes letting go during sex that much sweeter. If your partner isn't accustomed to taking the reins during sex, tell him frankly that you'd like for him to completely take things into his own hands the next time you are intimate. Tell him that you want him to have his way with you and to fulfill his every fantasy. Let him lead the way into a sexual experience that at other times you might say no to just because it would require you to release your control. Take a deep breath and truly submit.

WRITE IN DETAIL your experience with submission. Here are some questions to get you started: Have you ever submitted during sex? Do you enjoy being blindfolded? Bound? Do you like it rough? Do you like it when your partner takes control? If you have never experienced submission, what's stopping you?

"I want to live darkly and richly in my femaleness. I want a man lying over me, always over me. His will, his pleasure, his desire, his life, his work, his sexuality the touchstone, the command, my pivot." —ANAÏS NIN

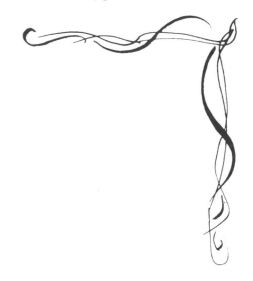

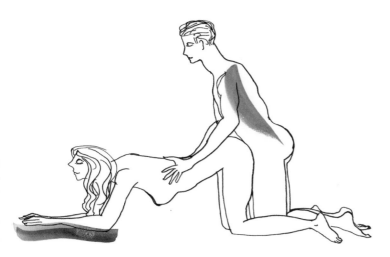

USING MARKERS, DRAW an image of what being sexually submissive means to you. You can make it as realistic or as abstract/symbolic as you like.

That Sexy Movie Scene

Have you ever been watching a regular Hollywood movie and found yourself to be completely, inexplicably (or maybe explicably) turned on? Use these pages to explore exactly what it is about a particular scene that you find so intoxicating.

FIRST GET YOUR HANDS on that movie and find the scene that arouses you. Now pretend you are the character in the movie scene and write out the scene in the first person, as if it happened to you. For example, maybe you play Kim Basinger's part in the iconic movie *9 1/2 Weeks* in the scene where Mickey Rourke is feeding her a myriad of sensual food items in the kitchen. You could write something like, "I was frightened when he told me to close my eyes—I didn't know what to expect! But then, when he put a sweet, red strawberry in my mouth and told me to bite down, I knew what kind of game we were playing." Have fun with it. Make your fantasy movie scene your fantasy reality!

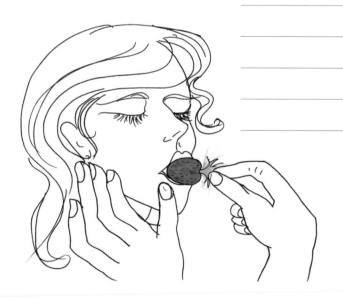

TAKE YOUR FAVORITE movie scene to the next level by role-playing with your partner. Try to capture as many details as possible, wear similar clothing as the characters in the movie, say the same lines, and reenact the sexy actions. Record your scene to watch later if that inspires you!

If role-playing with your partner makes you giggle a little, don't let that stop you! Getting playful and laughing in your sex life is only going to make it more fun.

Sex isn't supposed to be serious, steamy, and intense all the time. It can also be joyful, playful, and downright hilarious. Let go of your inhibitions, laugh a little, and have some fun!

Porn I Love

Porn is sexy, unapologetic, gritty, sleazy, exciting, boundary breaking, romantic, weird, titillating, and arousing, among many other things. Use these pages to explore your relationship with video porn.

WRITE DOWN YOUR EXPERIENCE WITH PORN. Here are some questions to get you started: How do you feel about pornography? Do you remember the first time you ever encountered pornographic material? How did you react? Have you ever found a porn video that really inspired you to push your own boundaries? What were the stand-out scenes? Write down any other feelings that you hold about porn.

Luckily, there are a lot of excellent pro-woman pornographers in the market today. For a great example of this, check out makelovenotporn.tv founded by Cindy Gallop. It's a crowd-sourced porn site that features real couples having real sex! The site is classy and safe, and five dollars gets you three weeks' access to a video; you also have the opportunity to share some of your own real sex videos, if that idea thrills the pants off of you.

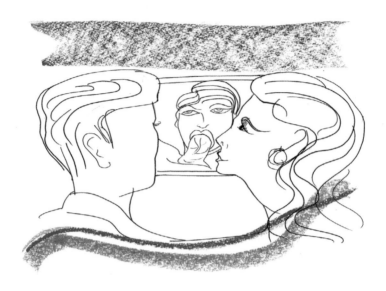

DRAW A PORN SCENE. Find a porn scene that really turns you on. (YouPorn.com has a variety of free videos to choose from.) Try masturbating to the video and notice when you climax. Return to that climactic moment in the film and pause the video. Using pencil, draw a copy of the stilled image. Take your time and try to really capture the scene. Next time you need a quick turn-on, you can refer to your drawing.

"Pornography is supposed to arouse sexual desires. If pornography is a crime, when will they arrest makers of perfume?"
—RICHARD FLEISCHER, AMERICAN FILM DIRECTOR

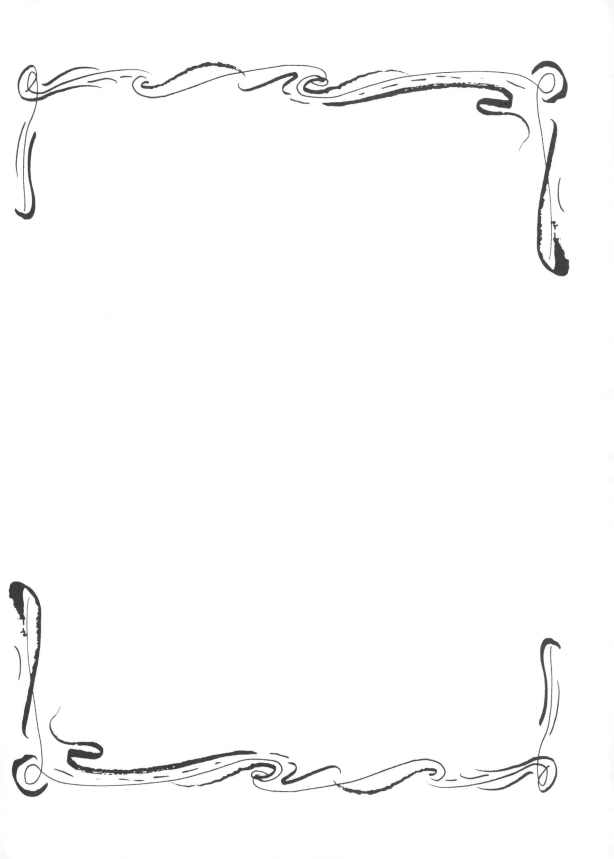

My Erotic Story

Erotica is a powerful tool of arousal. A well-written fantasy can stimulate your imagination and drive you to sensual heights. Use these pages to explore your erotic story.

WRITE YOUR OWN FANTASY erotica story. As you write your story, try filling in all of the following elements: What is the setting? Who are the characters? How do they meet? Why are they attracted to each other? How does the sexual tension build? How do they finally end up in bed together? How, exactly, does the sex play out? What happens after the sex act? Will the characters have a happy ending?

Erotica can be a great way to communicate your secret sexual desires with your partner. By writing your fantasy, you can express exactly what you want without coming right out and saying it. If you've wanted to explore bondage, or a threesome, or anal sex, or whatever it is, yet you're afraid to broach the topic, step into the waters of communication using erotica as your bridge. Judging by your partner's reaction to the story, you'll be able to tell whether your secret desire is something he or she would be interested in discussing and perhaps pursuing!

"Eros seizes and shakes my very soul / like the wind on the mountain / shaking ancient oaks." —SAPPHO, ANCIENT GREEK LYRIC POET

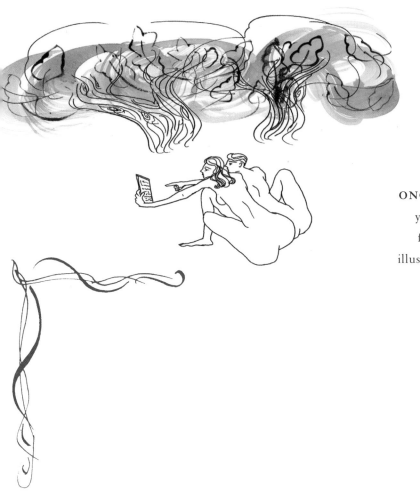

ONCE YOU'VE WRITTEN your erotic story, add some flare by offering your own illustrations to complement it.

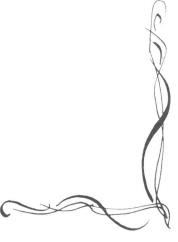

My (Fantasy) Sex Toy Collection

How many sex toys do you own? Is your secret bedside drawer overflowing? Do you only have a single favorite vibe? Or are you the type of woman who has never touched a sex toy in her life? Use these pages to explore your experience with adult toys.

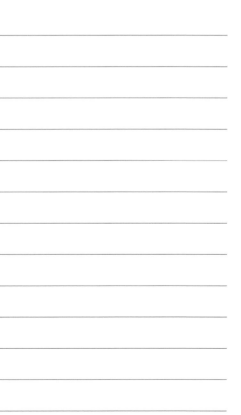

Are you shy about introducing a sex toy into your partnered sex? One of the best ways to incorporate the use of toys is by going shopping together (in a real store or online). By talking and thinking about the right purchase for you, you can learn a lot about each other's sexy ideas and begin building some new fantasies to share.

MAKE A LIST OF EVERY sex toy you own (or at least your favorites). In your list, include the reason that you like (or don't like) that particular toy. If you don't have many (or any!) toys, your challenge is to explore an online store and see if you can find any items that really pique your curiosity. Visit a safe and reputable site such as EdenFantasys.com or coco-de-mer.com to do some virtual window-shopping. Write down your fantasy sex toy list. You can later give it to your lover as a suggested gift list for your next birthday, holiday, or anniversary!

_____

_____

_____

_____

_____

_____

_____

_____

_____

_____

_____

_____

_____

MAKE YOUR OWN SEX TOY. Yes, it's true, for the crafty sex connoisseur, it's possible to make your own sex toy out of every-day items. If this is an art project that gets your juices flowing, visit the original DIY sex toy site homemade-sex-toys.com for a variety of fun XXX projects. Project ideas include the Frozen Cock-Sickle, which combines the best of the dildo and the Popsicle, or to practice sexy conservation, you might try making the DIY Solar-Powered Vibrator. Oh what fun!

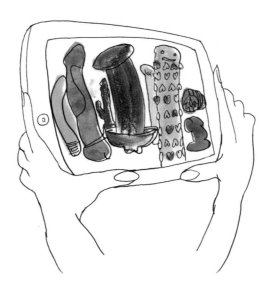

"The best sex I ever had was with my vibrator."
—EVA LONGORIA, AMERICAN ACTRESS

You Big Flirt!

Before the clothes ever hit the floor,
before the making out, even before
the dating comes the flirting.
Use these pages to explore your
experiences being a flirt.

WRITE DOWN WHAT
flirting means to you.
What's your secret flirting
maneuver? Write down a
scenario when you successfully flirted with someone and
include as much information
as you can recall. If you don't
consider yourself a flirt, why
aren't you? What's stopping
you? Do you think flirting
is useful or fun?

*"Some women flirt more with what they say, and
some with what they do."* —ANNA HELD,
EARLY TWENTIETH-CENTURY STAGE PERFORMER

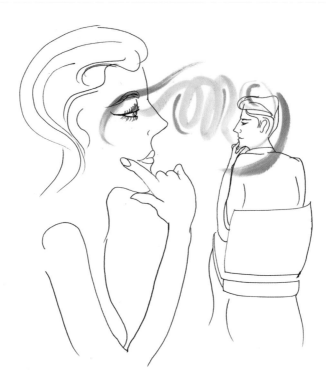

Here are six simple steps for successful flirting (and getting a date!):

1.

Make eye contact with your target. Let your eyes linger for a second before dropping them. If you meet your target's eyes, go to step two.

2.

Smile at your target. If your target smiles back, go to step three.

3.

Approach your target. This means you have to physically get into talking distance. If your target accepts your approach go to step four.

4.

Break the ice. Give your target a simple compliment like "I like your watch." If this successfully breaks the ice and you end up chatting, move to step five.

5.

Touch. Don't be too overt about it, but briefly touch his hand or wrist as you compliment him. If your target receives your touch positively, move to step six.

6.

Ask your target out. Ask your target if he or she would like to go have a cup of coffee with you sometime. If your target wants to upgrade your date offer to dinner, you have the option to accept or decline.

DRAW AN IMAGE of yourself being an amazing flirt. You can make this as abstract or realistic as you like.

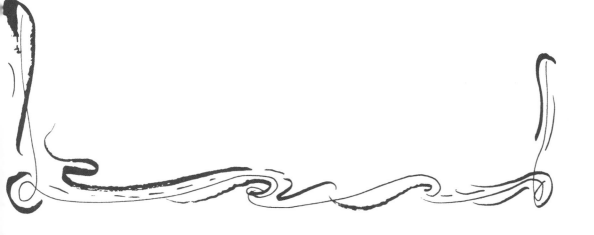

A Sexy Striptease

Sure, you get naked every morning and every evening, but have you ever slowed this down and turned it into a sexy striptease? Use these pages to explore your experience with taking your clothes off slowly and seductively.

WRITE DOWN YOUR experience with striptease: Have you ever performed an erotic striptease? What happened? Was it a public, private, professional, or drunken performance? Did you do it in front of a stranger, a lover, a friend? What was your audience's response? If you've never performed a striptease, why not? What's stopping you?

"If a thing is worth doing, it's worth doing slowly . . . very slowly."
—GYPSY ROSE LEE, AMERICAN BURLESQUE ENTERTAINER

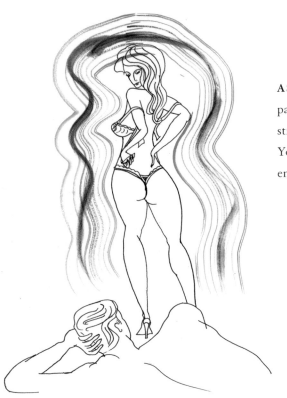

AS YOU PERFORM a striptease for your partner, have him take photos of you as you strip. Afterward, view them in sequence. You may be surprised at how sexy and empowered you look!

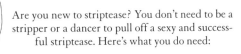

Are you new to striptease? You don't need to be a stripper or a dancer to pull off a sexy and successful striptease. Here's what you do need:

~

Confidence. It helps if you practice your performance a few times in front of a mirror before taking it live.

~

A sexy outfit that is easy to remove—for example, a silk robe, a pair of booty shorts, a bra, panties, and high heels.

~

A song that moves you.

~

No distractions. Put the pets and cell phones away.

~

Dim lights. They will make you feel sexier and less self-conscious. Moving slowly, remove each item of clothing in a teasing and seductive manner. Sway your hips. Touch your partner, but don't let him touch you . . . until you're ready!

Sex Tapes and Photos

Have you ever captured a sexy moment on camera? Use these pages to explore your experience with being the star of your own show.

WRITE ABOUT YOUR experience being in front of the camera. Think back to any times you've been photographed or taped while in a sexual situation. Here are some questions to get you started: What exactly were you doing and with whom? How did it make you feel to be taped while performing a sex act? If you've never been photographed or taped during sex, why not? Is this something that you would want to do?

_____

_____

_____

_____

_____

_____

_____

_____

_____

_____

_____

_____

_____

_____

_____

_____

TAKE A SEXY VIDEO or series of photos of you engaging in a sexual act with your partner. Try to remain anonymous in the video, showing only your body and not your face. Review the material later and choose your favorite scene or picture. Take the time to draw a pencil copy of this scene or picture and send it off in an unmarked envelope to your lover to enjoy.

"I always thought of photography as a naughty thing to do—that was one of my favorite things about it, and when I first did it, I felt very perverse."
—DIANE ARBUS, AMERICAN PHOTOGRAPHER

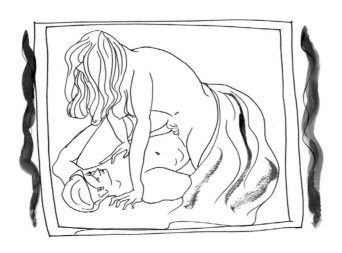

Real Sex / Fake Sex

In a culture nurtured on porn and Hollywood clichés, sometimes it can be hard to discern the difference between what is real and what is fake when it comes to sex. Use these pages to explore real sex versus fake sex.

WATCH A PORN FILM.

As you watch, write down anything that comes across as being inauthentic or implausible. Or maybe jot down some of the more ridiculous dialogue. Also write down anything that seems realistic or authentic. Maybe you happen upon a film where the woman is having a real orgasm and you can tell! By doing this writing exercise you can begin to pinpoint the differences between what is real and what is fake when it comes to performance sex.

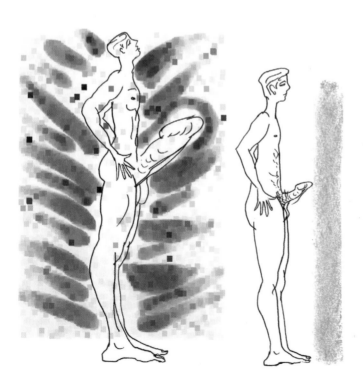

Don't feel bad if you enjoy the sensationalized version of sex that porn stars put into the world. The important thing is to remember that porn is not necessarily an accurate reflection of real sex. Porn is an exaggeration of the sexual experience, similar to how a circus performance, a blockbuster film, or a Broadway show is an exaggeration of the human experience.

DRAW TWO IMAGES side by side. In the first, draw an image that shows an exaggerated or fake version of sex. In the second, draw an image that shows an authentic or real version of sex. An example of this is drawing a porn star's penis beside that of your husband's, or a porn star's fake breasts beside your own. There are lots of possibilities.

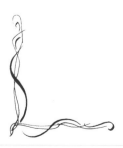

"My reaction to porno films is as follows: After the first ten minutes, I want to go home and screw. After the first twenty minutes, I never want to screw again as long as I live."

—ERICA JONG, AMERICAN AUTHOR

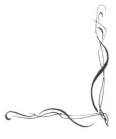

Morning Sex

Some women think that the morning is the most amazing time to have sex, while others find morning sex uncomfortable. Use these pages to explore your feelings about morning sex.

WHAT DOES MORNING
SEX MEAN TO YOU?
Write down your
responses to the following
leading sentences:

If you're in a relationship where finding time for sex is difficult and you often fall asleep as soon as your heads hit the pillows at night because of a trying day, having sex in the AM could be your solution. Morning sex is the one time when intimacy comes with pretty much zero baggage. You're relaxed, rested, and haven't yet been challenged, so it's the perfect opportunity to start your day off with a little pleasure!

I like morning sex when . . .

_____

_____

_____

The last time I had morning sex was. . .

_____

_____

_____

Morning sex makes me feel . . .

_____

_____

_____

My partner likes morning sex when . . .

_____

_____

_____

The best/worst thing about morning sex is . . .

_____

_____

_____

THE SOFT, EARLY morning light is one of the things that makes morning sex so enjoyable. Take advantage of the lighting and take a series of photos or make some drawings inspired by early morning loving.

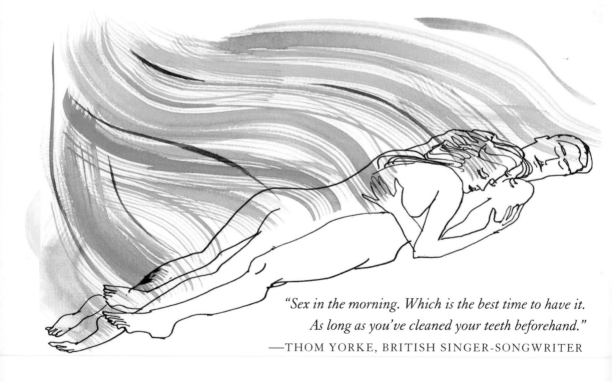

"Sex in the morning. Which is the best time to have it.
As long as you've cleaned your teeth beforehand."
—THOM YORKE, BRITISH SINGER-SONGWRITER

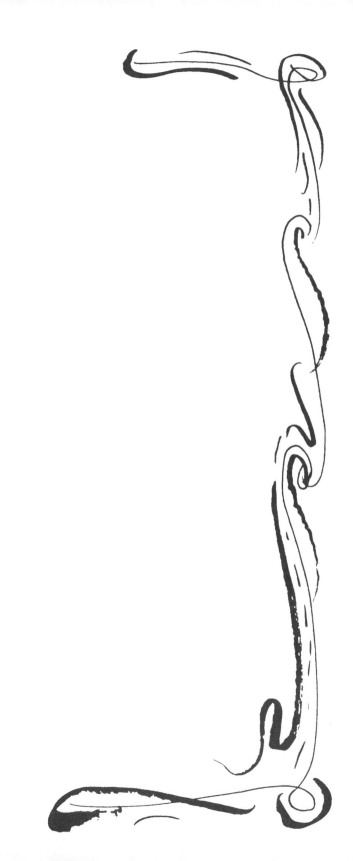

Nooners

Noon can feel like the naughtiest time of day to have sex. The middle of any given weekday is usually reserved for business meetings, running errands, or eating a microwave lunch in the employee kitchen. It is exceptionally sweet to be able to break away from the usual bustle of midday for some intimate time with your lover or yourself. Use these pages to explore your experience with nooners.

Make an explicit nooner date with your partner, or even with yourself, to add fun and excitement to your sex life. Plan a day where you and your partner can meet back home during your lunch break. (If home is too far, maybe meet at a cheap hotel or in the back of his work van!) Time will be of the essence—you both will probably have tasks to get back to—so enjoy the feeling of rushing through a quickie sex encounter and don't feel any pressure to achieve orgasm. You may find that the novelty of the situation is enough to get you off, but either way, you'll be heading back to your normal routine with a big smile on your face.

ENJOY A NOONER experience with yourself or your partner. Afterward, write down the experience in detail; include how it felt to go back to your usual day with that sexy interlude in the back of your mind.

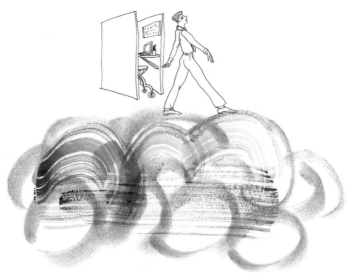

DRAW AN IMAGE of what midday sex means to you.
The image can be as realistic or as abstract as you want it to be.

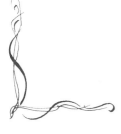

"Now I'm heading home for a nooner, which is what I call having pancakes for lunch." —LIZ LEMON, *30 ROCK*

My G-Spot

Have you found your G-spot yet? What has it done for you lately? Use these pages to explore your experience with stimulating your G-spot.

FIRST, LOCATE YOUR G-SPOT. It's located about one to three inches inside of your vagina, on the wall toward the front of your body. You'll know you have found it when you touch a spongy patch of tissue. Using your finger, stroke this spot and see what happens. After you've experimented, write down exactly how touching your G-spot made you feel. Use as much detail as possible. Did it feel pleasurable? Annoying? Exciting? Like nothing at all? Did it make you feel like you had to pee? Did it bring you to orgasm? Did you squirt? Is this something that you want to explore with your partner? Why or why not? If you're already familiar with your G-spot, describe exactly how G-spot stimulation makes you feel.

"What are you doing, trying to find my G-spot? Just stick it in! Go!" —JENKO, *21 JUMP STREET*

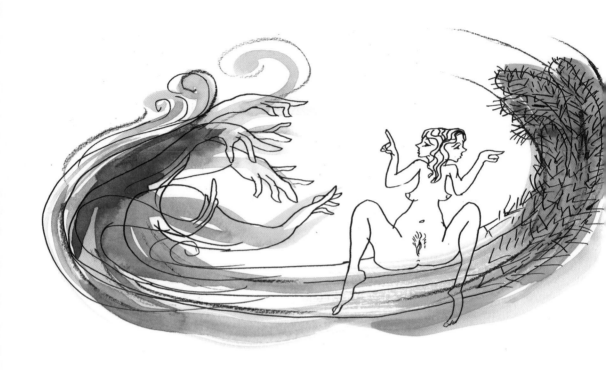

DRAW AN IMAGE of what you imagine your G-spot to look like. You can make this drawing as fanciful or as anatomical as you want. For example, if your G-spot frequently brings you to gushing orgasms, your image might be an ocean wave.

If rubbing your G-spot just annoys you, draw an image of it being like a prickly cactus. Have fun!

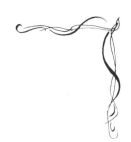
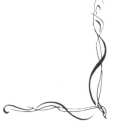

My Favorite (Go-To) Sex Position

There are some sex positions that are just so satisfying that it's easy to go back to them time and time again. Use these pages to explore your favorite sex positions.

WRITE DOWN YOUR TOP favorite sex positions. Include a reason why you would choose this to be your go-to position during intercourse—for example, "I love being on top during sex because I can rub my clitoris just right against my partner and have an orgasm every time." Or, "I love doggy style, the feeling of being dominated by my man while he is behind me is incomparable."

_____

_____

_____

_____

_____

_____

_____

_____

_____

_____

_____

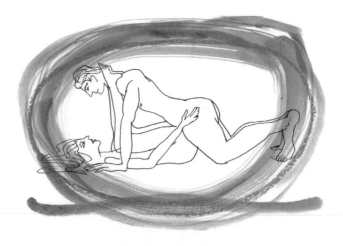

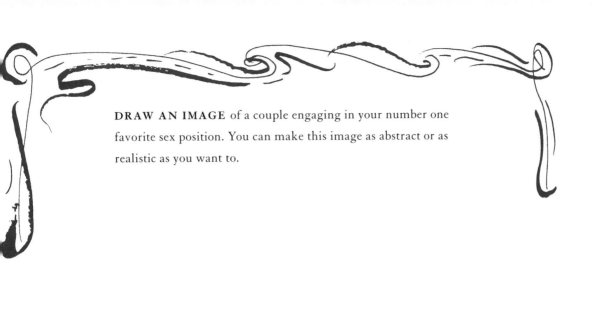

DRAW AN IMAGE of a couple engaging in your number one favorite sex position. You can make this image as abstract or as realistic as you want to.

Try a New Sex Position

When was the last time you tried out a new sex position? Use these pages to explore experimenting with something new.

WRITE DOWN A SCENARIO where you ended up in a new and exciting sex position. Describe how the position made you feel both physically and mentally. If you're not one who often explores new sex positions, describe a fantasy position that you'd like to try. Get into the detail of your memorable or fantastical new sex position and bring it to life on the page.

Are you looking for a new sex position to try? Sometimes all it takes is adding a little variation to a position that's tried and true. For example, in missionary position with him on top, rather than keeping your legs spread open, slide them closed and have him put his knees on either side of your thighs. This creates unbeatable friction as it squeezes your legs and pussy around his cock. For an extensive list of position ideas, visit WeWomen.com/relationships and search for "sex positions."

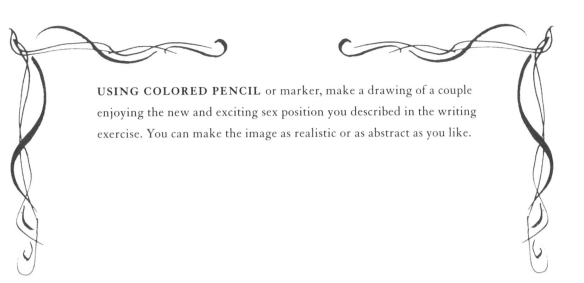

USING COLORED PENCIL or marker, make a drawing of a couple enjoying the new and exciting sex position you described in the writing exercise. You can make the image as realistic or as abstract as you like.

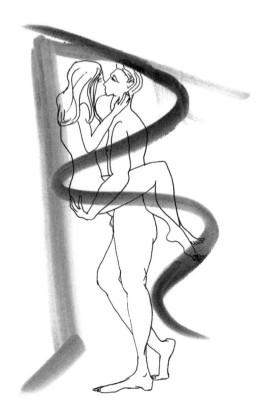

Losing My Virginity

Losing your virginity is something that can only happen once. Often our culture builds it up to be such a momentous occasion and important rite of passage that the actual event itself can leave you feeling confused, disappointed, or worse. Use these pages to explore your personal experience with losing your virginity.

What does it really mean for a woman to lose her virginity? In the United States, the more traditional definition is that losing your virginity requires sexual penetration by a penis. But what if your first sexual encounter is with another woman? What if she penetrates you with finger or toy? For this reason, it makes sense to define losing your virginity as happening the first time you reveal your sexuality to another person, the first time you undress, caress, and become truly intimate with someone else.

IN DETAIL, WRITE ABOUT your first sexual experience. Here are some questions to get you started: Who was your first? Where were you? How did it feel? How old were you? What were your hopes and fears for the situation? Who was your first real lover—was it the same person as who you lost your virginity to? Were you surprised? Disappointed? Confused? Delighted? In love? Satisfied?

_____

_____

_____

_____

_____

_____

_____

"I lost my virginity when I was fourteen. And I haven't been able to find it." —DAVID DUCHOVNY, AMERICAN ACTOR

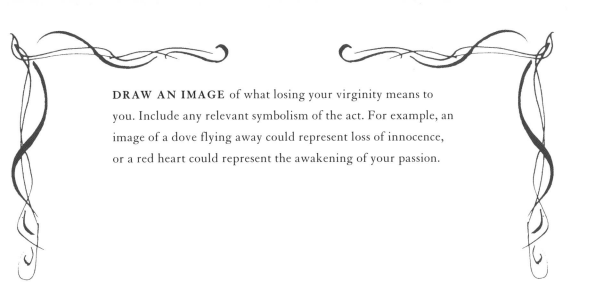

DRAW AN IMAGE of what losing your virginity means to you. Include any relevant symbolism of the act. For example, an image of a dove flying away could represent loss of innocence, or a red heart could represent the awakening of your passion.

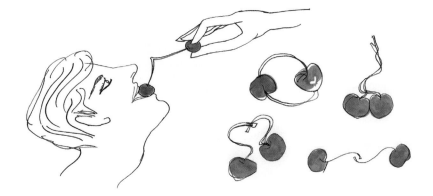

My First Time with My Current Partner

Do you remember the first time you had sex with your current partner? Use these pages to delve into this encounter.

THINK ABOUT THE first time you had sex with your current (or your most recent or most impactful) lover. Write down, in detail, the circumstances of this encounter. Here are some questions to get you started: How long had you known your partner before having sex? How did it feel to have sex for the first time? Exciting? Electric? Romantic? Gentle? Ferocious? Did you have an orgasm? Where were you when the encounter happened? What was the mood? Add any other details you can remember about this experience.

If you've been in a relationship for a while, you may find that your sex life needs some of the excitement of the first time. Play a little game of Strangers at a Bar. Arrange to meet your partner at a predetermined location, but arrive separately. Upon seeing your partner, start a conversation with him or her that makes it seem as if you two are strangers. Allow the interaction to happen as if it's the first time, and flirt your way into a romantic and sexy situation. You can even use alternate names or wear a wig to make the game seem more realistic.

_____

_____

_____

_____

_____

_____

_____

_____

_____

_____

_____

_____

_____

_____

_____

_____

_____

_____

_____

"Whenever a thing is done for the first time, it releases a little demon." —EMILY DICKINSON, AMERICAN POET

MAKE A COMIC STRIP
that illustrates your first encounter with your current, most recent, or most impactful partner. Illustrate your meeting, your first kiss, and how you ended up in a sexual tryst—make it as romantic or as sexy as you want to. If drawing a comic strip is a little out of your comfort zone, visit Chogger.com and make one using their fun, online tool that allows you to pick a layout, upload photos or make digital drawings, and insert speech balloons!

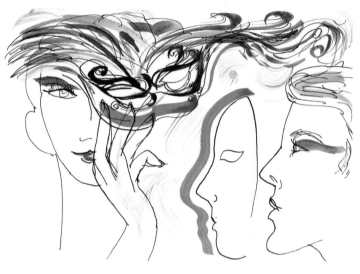

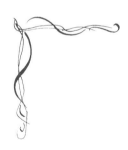
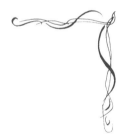
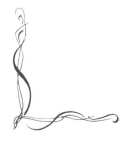
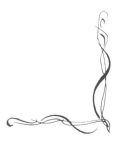

My First (Fantasy) Threesome

Have you ever been in a threesome, foursome, or moresome? Have you ever wanted to try? Use these pages to explore your first threesome, or if you've never been in one, explore your fantasy ménage à trois.

DESCRIBE IN DETAIL your first (or fantasy) threesome. Who were your two partners? What sexual games did you play? What was your role in the threesome? Were you an active participant? Were you submissive or dominant? Were you a voyeur on the sidelines? Was it romantic, depraved, exciting—something else? How did you feel during the encounter? How did you feel when the encounter was over? Would you participate in another threesome with these partners? Would you pursue a threesome with another trio? If so, who?

To avoid jealousy or complications, it's a good idea to go into a threesome with some relationship rules. Talk about how you'll choose a third partner and how you both have the power to veto a third partner at any time in the process. Decide whether you'd like for it to be a stranger or someone you know. Decide in advance what activities you are allowed to participate in with your third partner (e.g., kissing, penetration, cuddling). If you're not seeking a polyamorous relationship but are more interested in having a singular experience, it's best to engage in a threesome in a city that's not your hometown.

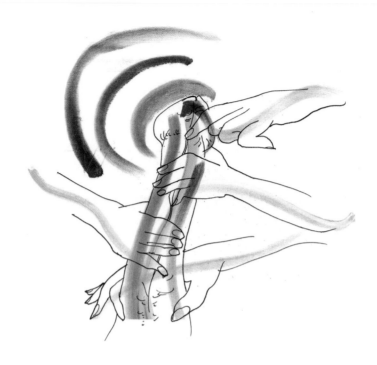

DRAW AN IMAGE of a threesome sexual encounter.
Make it as realistic or as abstract as you like.

Bret: Have you ever had a threesome?

Jemaine: Nearly.

Bret: What do you mean "nearly"?

Jemaine: I've had a twosome.
—BRET MCKENZIE AND JEMAINE CLEMENT,
    FLIGHT OF THE CONCHORDS

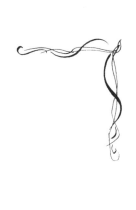
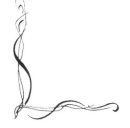

Past Experiences

Your sex life makes up part of your unique human experience. Often, past sexual experiences are locked up in the deepest corners of your memories and never paid any attention to, or worse, cloaked in shame and regret. By taking out and inspecting your past sexual experiences just as you would an old picture album, you can learn more about yourself and your desires and begin to understand what turns you on and what makes you wholly human.

Sharing your past experiences with your present partner can be exciting and can open up new doors to communication and sexual exploration. If you or your partner feel a little shy about sharing, play a game of "I'll share with you, if you share with me." Using the writing exercise in this section, both of you write down one of your most memorable past experiences on a piece of paper and then exchange it with each other. Read your partner's experience aloud to him, and have him read yours aloud to you. Take this a step further by re-creating (or fantasizing about re-creating) the experience together!

WRITE ABOUT YOUR most vivid sexual experience, who was there? Where were you? What were you doing? How did it feel?

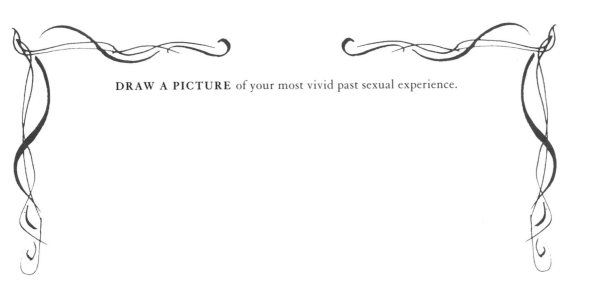

DRAW A PICTURE of your most vivid past sexual experience.

"We are all born sexual creatures, thank God, but it's a pity so many people despise and crush this natural gift." —MARILYN MONROE

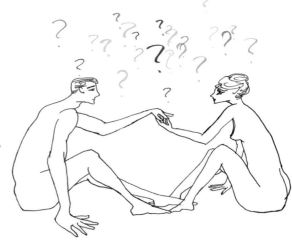

My Most Memorable Lover

Most women have a specific lover who, no matter what else happens in their sex lives, is truly unforgettable. It could be your first true love; it could be the lifeguard with the big, beautiful penis; or it could be the bad boy who crushed your heart but delivered hundreds of orgasms during your tumultuous time together. Use these pages to explore your most memorable lover.

If you are no longer with your most memorable lover, it's important to leave the past in the past. If you find yourself comparing your current lover with the one you lost, you may discover that you're not enjoying your present day sex life as much as is possible. Start building new memories with your present-day lover. A fun exercise is to write down a couple of things every day that your current lover does that make you feel amazing.

DESCRIBE IN DETAIL your most memorable lover. Who was he or she? What makes him or her memorable? Was it the way he touched you? Was it the way he looked? Was it the way she treated you? Describe some of your most exciting sexual experiences together.

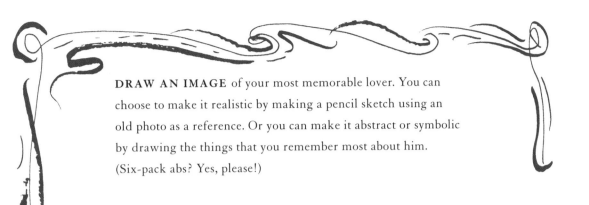

DRAW AN IMAGE of your most memorable lover. You can choose to make it realistic by making a pencil sketch using an old photo as a reference. Or you can make it abstract or symbolic by drawing the things that you remember most about him. (Six-pack abs? Yes, please!)

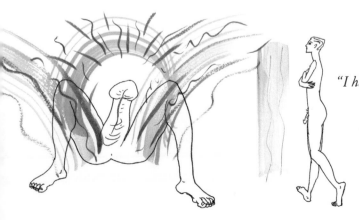

"I have tried to let you go and I cannot. I cannot stop thinking of you. I cannot stop dreaming about you."
—ERIN MORGENSTERN,
THE NIGHT CIRCUS

That Wild Time

Have you ever experienced a time in your life when you were particularly open to sexual exploration and pushing the boundaries of inhibitions? Use these pages to explore the situations when you've let your hair down and gone a little (or a lot!) wild in your sex life.

THINK BACK TO A TIME in your life when you felt uninhibited and wildly sexy. Maybe it was your senior year at university when you and your roommate made an unabashed game of reeling in guys for threesomes. Maybe your wild time happened after your divorce when you began to explore your inner sex diva and prowled the bars for new blood. Maybe it started in your forties when you and your partner decided to explore swinging. Whatever the circumstances, describe the wilder things you've done in your sex life. Who were you with? What exactly happened? Given the opportunity, would you behave this way again? Why or why not?

If your wild days included experiences with a lot of new partners but now you are in a committed relationship, talk to your partner about ways to incorporate this bit of inhibition safely into your sex life. This could take the form of watching porn featuring group sex, teaming up with your partner to have sexy chats with strangers online, or maybe even visiting a sex club and watching other people getting busy (or letting them watch you!). It's up to you how much to let the wild back in!

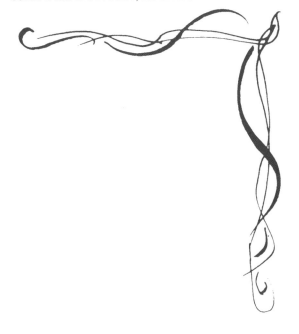

"You were once wild here. Don't let them tame you."
—ISADORA DUNCAN, AMERICAN DANCER

DRAW WHAT "being uninhibited" means to you. You could depict an image of something as innocent as flashing your boobs at Mardi Gras, or as naughty as engaging in bukkake.

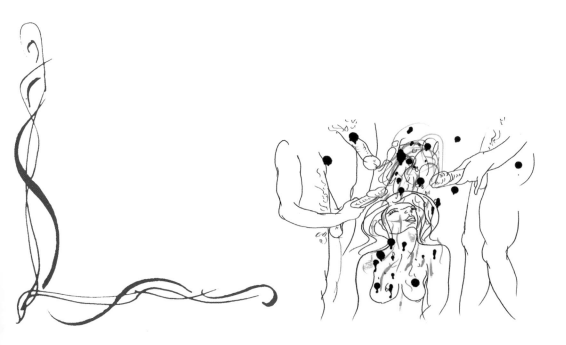

I'm a Sexpert At...

You know you're damn good at something when it comes to sex. Use these pages to explore your own inner sexpert.

THINK BACK TO compliments that your partner(s) has given you. Have you been praised for your blow job, extolled for your hand job, or given accolades for your flexibility during intercourse? When it comes to sex, what do you pride yourself for being really, truly good at? Describe how you came to be an expert at this one particular thing and how giving this sex act to your partner makes you feel.

_____

_____

_____

_____

_____

_____

_____

_____

_____

_____

_____

_____

_____

_____

_____

_____

_____

_____

_____

_____

GIVE EACH OTHER a medal! Use Snapguide.com's "How to Make a Paper Medal" tutorial to create an award to honor yourself for your sexpertise and your partner's for his! Be sure to write what your award is for, whether it's Best Blow Job or Most Impressive Dominatrix. Give each other the award, and then hang the medals in your closet or somewhere that only you and your intimate partner will see them; they are sure to give you a smile every time you get a glimpse and perhaps will inspire you to action.

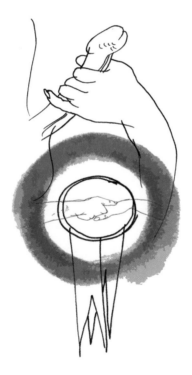

"Try, try, try, and keep on trying is the rule that must be followed to become an expert in anything."
—W. CLEMENT STONE,
AMERICAN AUTHOR AND PHILANTHROPIST

Sex Guilt

Has having sex or sexual desires ever made you feel guilty? Use these pages to explore the concept of sex guilt.

WRITE ABOUT YOUR SEX GUILT. Do you ever feel guilty about your sexual desires? If so, which desires in particular make you feel the most shamed? Where did you learn to feel guilty about sex? Do you think that there is a right way and a wrong way to have sex? If yes, where does this belief come from? Is there something that would help you feel less guilty? Do you feel you need approval from someone or something?

Feelings of guilt and shame can be directly related to feelings of arousal. When a sex act makes you feel like you are crossing into the taboo, it can have that much more appeal. For example, exploring anal sex may make you feel like you are doing something naughty, unnatural, or wrong, which heightens the feelings of satisfaction that you gain from the act. For this reason, next time you feel shameful about a sex act you are participating in, turn that feeling of guilt into a feeling of decadent satisfaction. So long as your actions are safe, sane, and consensual, you have the right to explore your body to its fullest—guilty feelings and all.

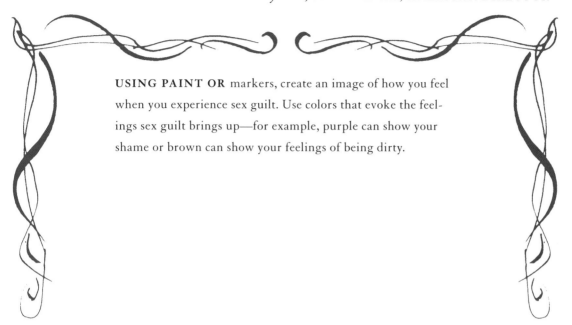

"I thank God I was raised Catholic, so sex will always be dirty." —JOHN WATERS, AMERICAN DIRECTOR

USING PAINT OR markers, create an image of how you feel when you experience sex guilt. Use colors that evoke the feelings sex guilt brings up—for example, purple can show your shame or brown can show your feelings of being dirty.

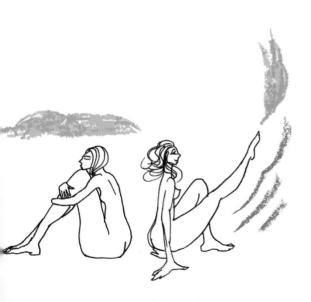

Sometimes When I'm Fucking I Think About. . .

You're in the middle of having good,
maybe even *great*, sex when—**poof**—
suddenly, out of nowhere, a totally
random thought comes to mind.
What do you sometimes catch
yourself thinking about during sex?
Use these pages to explore those intruder thoughts.

When you catch yourself thinking about something besides the sexy
moment you are in, use this process to center your thoughts and
bring them back to the sensations at hand.

~

Replace the intruder thought with an observation about a physical
sensation that you are having in the moment. If you are having
trouble focusing on what's happening now, do a scan of your body,
starting with how your toes are feeling, then moving up your legs, and
higher and higher. What is that tingling sensation you are feeling in
your lower belly? By focusing on the sensations you are feeling, you'll
be able to bring your mind back to the present sexual experience.

THINK BACK TO THOSE moments when your mind wandered during sex. Write the thoughts down, sparing no details. Allowing a place for those thoughts to play will give them less power. Do you notice a theme? Is your mind consumed by daily chores or work? Is it consumed by past experiences, or by how you are performing in bed? Or are you thinking about something you wish your lover was doing, but he's not?

_____

_____

_____

_____

_____

_____

_____

_____

_____

_____

_____

_____

_____

_____

_____

_____

DRAW A SKETCH of some of the most common distractions that pop up during sex. For example, sketch a pile of dirty laundry if your pillowcases are driving you to distraction. Now take a fat black marker and draw a thick *X* over each distraction that you've drawn. Next time you are having sex, picture drawing a thick, black *X* over any thoughts that intrude on your good time.

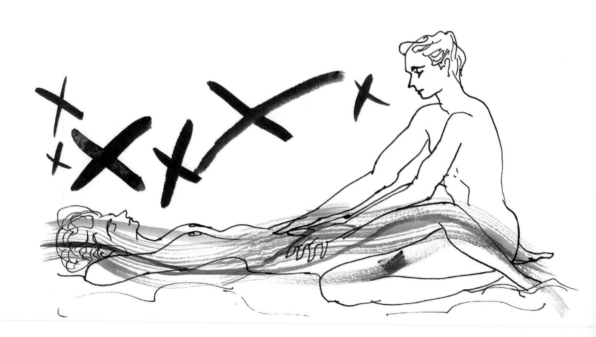

"Be master of mind rather than mastered by mind." —ZEN PROVERB

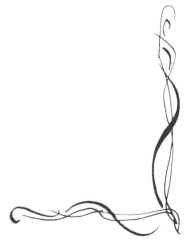

My Perception Of Sex Changed When . . .

Do you remember when your perception of sex changed? Use these pages to explore the pivotal times in your life that altered your views on what sex is all about.

HAVE YOU EVER HAD a partner or experience that completely transformed your perception of sex? Maybe you went from a long-term, vanilla marriage into a whirlwind relationship with a sexually adventurous man. Or maybe you went from a traditional religion, believing that sex is sacred to a husband and wife, to the pagan experience of sex being natural and free. Or maybe you discovered that you prefer the soft kiss of a woman to the rough touch of a man. Write down those moments in your life where your idea of sex was flipped on its head. What happened? Who or what inspired the change? Offer as much detail as possible.

"There is no truth, only perception."
—GUSTAVE FLAUBERT, FRENCH NOVELIST

MIRROR IMAGES. On one half of the page, draw an image of what sex meant to you *before* your pivotal moment. On the other half, draw an image of what your definition of sex became *after* this moment. For example, on one side you could draw a man and a woman engaged in romantic love, and on the other, you could draw a woman surrounded by a circle of aroused men.

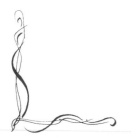

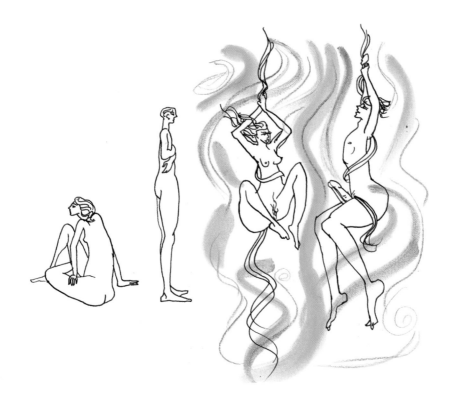

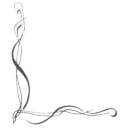
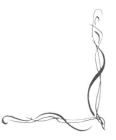

Faking It

There are many reasons why women may fake an orgasm. Faking it can be a way for a woman to end a dissatisfying sexual experience, or to satisfy a partner's ego. Use these pages to explore your experience with faking it.

WRITE DOWN YOUR experience with faking orgasms. Use these questions to get you started: Have you ever faked an orgasm? Why or why not? How does faking an orgasm make you feel in the end? Do you feel like faking it is worth it? Do you have difficulty achieving orgasm in partnered sex? How about during masturbation? If your partner found out you faked it, what do you think he or she would do?

Although you may have some very compelling reasons to fake an orgasm, by faking it you end up miseducating your partner and short-changing yourself. It's okay for you to not have an orgasm every single time you are intimate, but it's not okay to tell your partner that he is reliably bringing you to orgasm when he's not. If you've been faking it for a while, you're going to have to fess up. Only then can you and your partner start collaborating on ways to truly bring you to bliss.

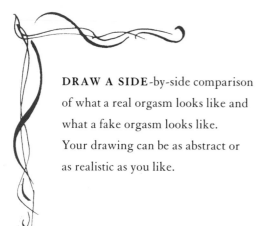

DRAW A SIDE-by-side comparison
of what a real orgasm looks like and
what a fake orgasm looks like.
Your drawing can be as abstract or
as realistic as you like.

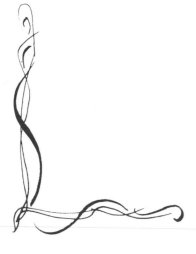

"You know there are two types of female orgasm: the real and the fake. And I'll tell you right now, as a man, we don't know. We do not know, because to man sex is like a car accident and determining the female orgasm is like being asked, 'What did you see after the car went out of control?' 'I heard a lot of screeching sounds. I remember I was facing the wrong way at one point. And in the end my body was thrown clear.'"

—JERRY SEINFELD, AMERICAN COMEDIAN

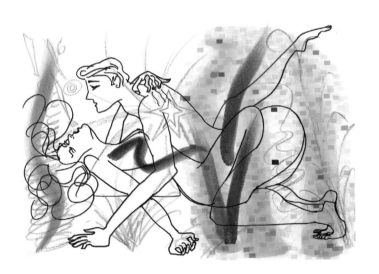

Phone Sex

Has your partner ever been away for a business trip and you felt just completely out of your skin horny for him or her? Did you pick up the phone? Use these pages to explore your experiences with phone sex.

WRITE DOWN DIALOGUE of a phone sex conversation that you have had or would love to have with your partner. Be explicit and spare no detail.

_____

_____

_____

_____

_____

_____

_____

_____

_____

_____

_____

_____

_____

_____

_____

_____

_____

_____

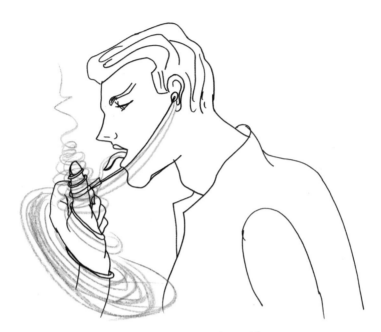

RECORD AN EXPLICIT conversation with your partner. (There are many smartphone apps you can use to do this with, including Google Voice.) Trim down the call to just its most essential and sexy elements. Over time, send your partner snippets of the conversation in the form of electronic love notes.

"Humans are the only animal who can have sex over the phone." —DAVID LETTERMAN, AMERICAN COMEDIAN AND LATE-NIGHT TALK SHOW HOST

Dirty Talk

When done well, dirty talk can be the spice of your sex life. A well-placed dirty word or a bit of provocative name calling can be a thigh-tingling experience. Use these pages to explore your experience with the art of dirty talk.

Some people may feel a little shy talking dirty in the bedroom. If you or your partner have a hard time uttering filthy phrases in each other's ears but have the desire to hear these naughty phrases said aloud, try reading particularly raunchy erotic poems and stories to each other. By reading someone else's words, you'll be removing the responsibility for what you're saying from your own conscience, yet still have the luxury of talking dirty to your partner.

WRITE DOWN A LIST of at least ten naughty names that you would like your partner to call you during sex. For example, "bad girl," "cum slut," "sex goddess," or "mistress." Now write down a list of at least ten dirty phrases that you like to hear in bed. This could include phrases such as "Bend over the bed" or "Let me see your pussy," or whatever phrases come to mind that really get your motor running. If you're feeling bold, share these lists with your partner.

CREATE A DIRTY-talk collage. Using text from magazines or the Web, cut out letters and words to create a collage of dirty words and phrases that turn you on. You can spice up the collage by including erotically charged images, too.

"For women the best aphrodisiacs are words. The G-spot is in the ears. He who looks for it below there is wasting his time."
—ISABEL ALLENDE, CHILEAN AUTHOR

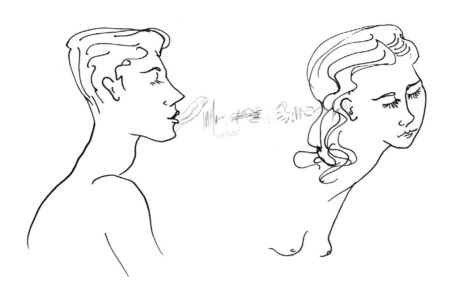

An Aural Sex Poem

Take the art of dirty talk to the next level by creating your very own aural sex poem. Use these pages to write an erotic poem.

A SIMPLE WAY TO WRITE an erotic poem is to capture the real images and feelings that transpire during sex. Start out by jotting down a few stand-out images that come up during your next several intimate moments. An example could be "Your hand on my thigh, your skin so dark against mine so pale." Or maybe "The lust burning in your eyes" or "The sting of your palm on my skin as you spank me." Once you've got a list of strong images from your encounters, you can weave them together into a full-length poem. Write your aural sex poem here. Remember it doesn't have to rhyme, be any specific length, or be publication ready, but hopefully it arouses and inspires your erotic experience. If you feel brave, read your poem aloud to your partner while wearing something sexy.

"Poetry is the art of uniting pleasure with truth."
—SAMUEL JOHNSON, EIGHTEENTH CENTURY ENGLISH WRITER

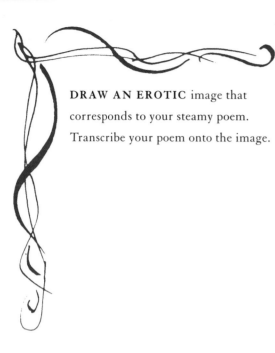

DRAW AN EROTIC image that
corresponds to your steamy poem.
Transcribe your poem onto the image.

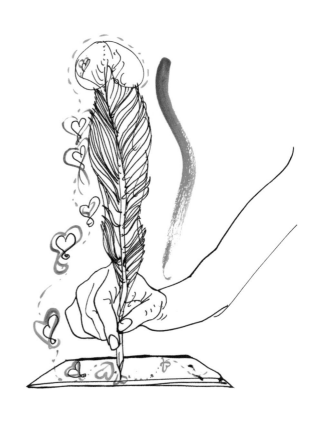

One-Night Stands

A one-night stand can be quite the sexy adventure; it's an intimate moment with the exotically intoxicating presence of a nearly complete stranger or a friend who you never thought you'd be with *in that way.* Use these pages to explore your experiences with one-night stands.

HAVE YOU EVER HAD a one-night stand, a single instance of sexual pleasure with a friend or stranger? Who was it with? What were the circumstances surrounding the encounter? What did you do together? How did you feel about the encounter the next day? In general, how do you feel about one-night stands?

If you think there's even a chance that you might ever, ever engage in a one-night stand, always bring your own condoms. Because you are exchanging very personal fluids with someone you don't know all that well, the need to use protection is that much more imperative. For some stylish, eco-friendly, and socially responsible condoms, visit sirrichards.com; for every condom you buy from them, they donate one to a developing country.

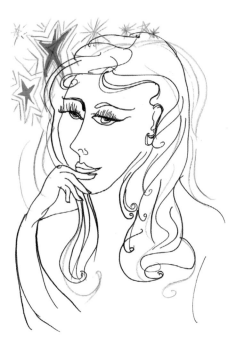

DRAW AN IMAGE of how a one-night stand makes you feel, using colors and shapes that best express the emotions that you are left with. For example, black circles might indicate emptiness, or hot-pink stars might express your wildness.

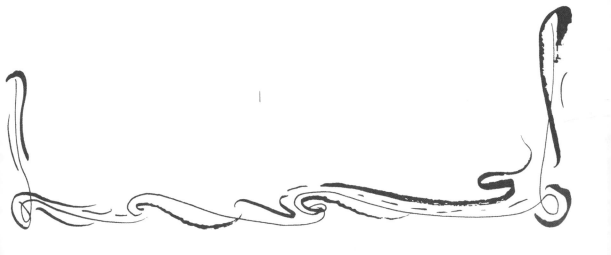

Exploring My Sexual Power

Many women spend a lot of time working on their appearance, careers, parenting skills, friendships, and other areas of life. But what about manifesting your sexual power? Use these pages to uncover what makes you an undeniably sexy goddess.

THINK BACK TO TIMES in your life when you felt really sexy and sensual. What exactly contributed to this feeling of power? Was it when you rendered your partner helpless after an unbeatable blow job? Or was it when you walked into a room and you knew that you could have your choice of partners? Describe any time that you felt truly sexually empowered. If you've never felt sexually empowered, try describing what is holding you back. What are some negative beliefs you have about your sexuality that you'd need to let go of in order to manifest your true sex goddess?

"If you realized how powerful your thoughts are, you would never think a negative thought."
—PEACE PILGRIM, AMERICAN PEACE ACTIVIST

DRAW YOURSELF as an all-powerful sex goddess. Pay attention to how being a sex goddess would show up in your appearance and also in your inner power and stature. Use colors and shapes that embody the feelings of the sexual power that you would possess. The image can be as abstract or as realistic as you like.

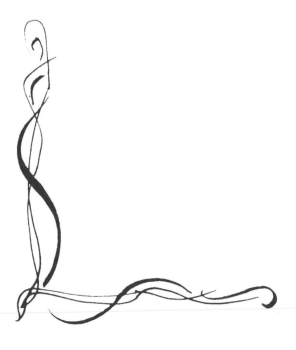

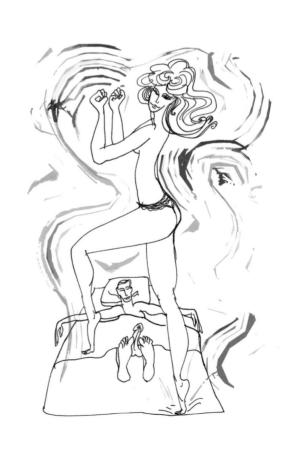

I Have (Never) Cheated . . .

Have you ever cheated
on a partner? Have
you ever been cheated
on? Use these pages to
explore your experience
with cheating.

THINK BACK TO AN experience you've
had with cheating or being cheated on. Write
about the events that took place. How did
cheating make you feel? Was it worth it?
What did you learn from the experience? How
has your experience with cheating affected
your current relationship? Do you believe that
monogamy can work? Why or why not?

_____

_____

_____

_____

_____

_____

_____

_____

_____

_____

_____

_____

_____

_____

_____

_____

_____

_____

_____

"Heartbreak is good fuel for country songs. And cheating."
—MIRANDA LAMBERT, AMERICAN COUNTRY MUSIC ARTIST

USING PAINT OR markers, create an image of how cheating makes you feel. Use colors that evoke the feelings that come up. For example, black could show your anger, while red could show passion or excitement.

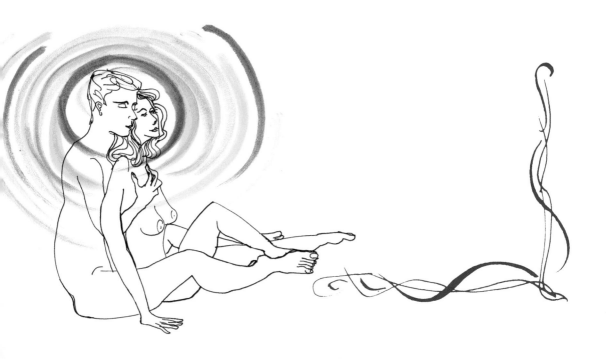

The Notches in My Bedpost

All right, tell the truth! How many people have you slept with in your lifetime? In these pages, take a look at the notches in your personal bedpost.

WRITE DOWN THE FIRST NAME (or initials) of every lover you've ever had (or at least, every lover you can remember!). Then write down a brief, one-sentence memory of each encounter. Here's an example: *Gabriel the Cuban—I was attracted to him because of how good he smelled. He ended up having the nicest model body and a big, yummy cock!*

_____

_____

_____

_____

_____

_____

_____

_____

_____

_____

_____

_____

_____

_____

_____

_____

"You know, my bedpost really has very few notches compared with other actors of my erm, erm, pedigree."
— DAVID TENNANT, SCOTTISH ACTOR

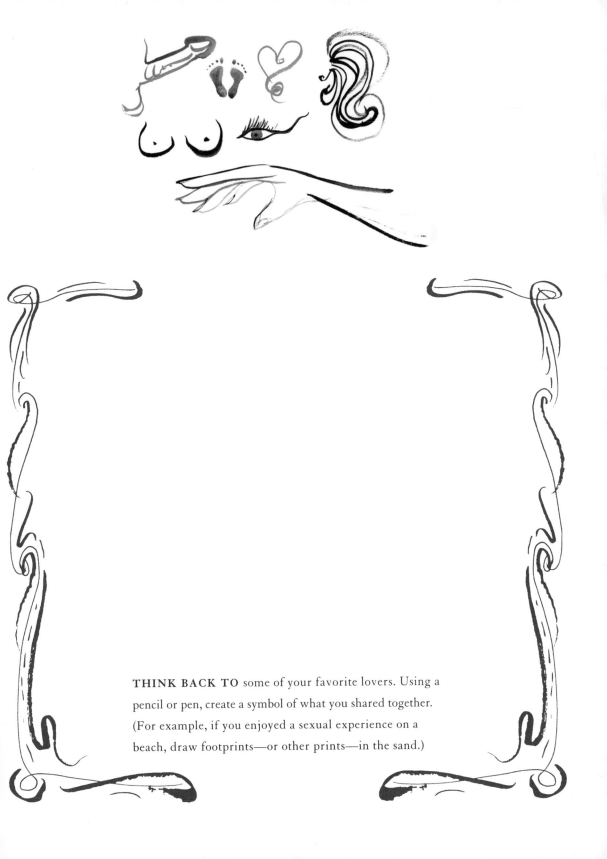

THINK BACK TO some of your favorite lovers. Using a pencil or pen, create a symbol of what you shared together. (For example, if you enjoyed a sexual experience on a beach, draw footprints—or other prints—in the sand.)

About the Author

Jordan LaRousse is the co-author of *Penis Genius*,
Clit-ology, and *Mastering Your Man from Head to Head*
and the co-editor of two erotic anthologies.
She believes that great sex comes from
that spark when the mind, body, and imagination
come together in perfect harmony.

© 2014 Quiver
Illustrations © 2014 Margaret Hurst

First published in the USA in 2014 by
Quiver, a member of
Quarto Publishing Group USA Inc.
100 Cummings Center
Suite 406-L
Beverly, MA 01915-6101
www.quiverbooks.com

18 17 16 15 14   1 2 3 4 5

ISBN: 978-1-59233-611-1

Cover and book design by The Lincoln Avenue Workshop
Illustrations by Margaret Hurst

Printed and bound in Hong Kong